INDIVIDUALS IN CONTEXT

A Practical Guide to Client-Centered Practice

Edited by

Virginia G. Fearing, BSc(OT), OT(C), OTR
Jo Clark, BSc(OT), OT(C)
Vancouver Hospital & Health Sciences Centre
Vancouver, British Columbia, Canada

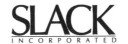

SLACK
I N C O R P O R A T E D

6900 Grove Road, Thorofare, NJ 08086

Publisher: John H. Bond
Editorial Director: Amy E. Drummond

On cover: Occupational Performance Process Model from Fearing, V.G., Law, M., & Clark, J. (1997). An occupational performance process model: Fostering client and therapist alliances. *Canadian Journal of Occupational Therapy, 64*, 11. Reprinted with permission of CAOT Publications.
Cover idea by Jenna Clark (age 11).

The work SLACK publishes is peer reviewed. Prior to publication, recognized leaders in the field, educators, and clinicians provide important feedback on the concepts and content that we publish. We welcome feedback on this book.

Individuals in context : a practical guide to client-centered practice / edited by Virginia G. Fearing, Jo Clark.
    p. ; cm.
    Includes bibliographical references and index.
    ISBN: 1-55642-417-5 (alk paper)
    1. Occupational therapy. 2. Client-centered psychotherapy. 3. Medical personnel and patient. I. Fearing, Virginia G. (Virginia Griswold). II. Clark, Jo.
    [DNLM: 1. Occupational therapy--methods. 2. Patient-Centered Care. 3. Professional-Patient Relations. WB 555 I39 2000]
    RM735.4 .I53 2000
    616.89'14--dc21   00-030070

Printed in the United States of America.

Published by: SLACK Incorporated
                6900 Grove Road
                Thorofare, NJ 08086-9447 USA
                Telephone: 856-848-1000
                Fax: 856-853-5991
                www.slackbooks.com

Contact SLACK Incorporated for more information about other books in this field or about the availability of our books from distributors outside the United States.

Last digit is print number: 10 9 8 7 6 5 4 3 2 1

DEDICATION

This book is dedicated to occupational therapists all over the world.
May it help you better understand and put into practice what you already know.

The mind is not a vessel to be filled,
but a fire to be kindled.
(Plutarch)

CONTENTS

(S) SAFEWAY

CANADA SAFEWAY
GST #R119347672

GEN MERCHANDISE

HLMK VAL CARD WW		.99 GP
**** 7.0% GST DUE		.07
**** 7.0% PST DUE		.07
**** TAX	.14 BAL	1.13
CASH		1.25

CHANGE .12
NUMBER OF ITEMS = 1
2/11/05 12:27 0028 03 0062 7306

ACKNOWLEDGMENTS

The editors are indebted to the contributing authors, who speak so eloquently regarding client-centered practice and who managed, in spite of living in contexts that included birth, death, injury, layoff, hospitalization, and heavy workloads, to meet deadlines with grace and humor.

We are grateful to the hundreds of occupational therapists whose open sharing and thoughtful comments at workshops over the past 10 years have enriched our thinking. Thank you Mary Clark Green, Westprint Communications, for the early graphic work on the Occupational Performance Process Model and Paul Fearing for the tireless hours spent on the rendition found in this book. Dr. Mary Ferguson-Paré, Vice-President of Professional Affairs, Vancouver Hospital & HSC, gave us courage through her belief in client-centered practice, in us, and in this book.

The gift of Shirley Salomon's time, support, and excitement as she carefully read the complete manuscript is appreciated and has made a positive difference in the clarity of the content. Discussions with Julie Stockton, who read portions of the manuscript, were invaluable. Thank you Mary Law for your support and encouragement. We consider ourselves fortunate to be occupational therapists and working among such fine colleagues.

To the editors of SLACK Incorporated, Amy Drummond, Debra Toulson, and Kate Buczko: Thank you for believing in us and for helping make this book a reality.

We wish to thank our families: Harold and Paul Fearing and Steve, Ty, and "Wigs" Clark. It is wonderful to live in homes filled with love. And finally, thank you to our parents Marvel and Ernest Griswold (both deceased) and Doris and Henry Buckles, whose values, including continuous learning, have certainly shaped our own and, therefore, are echoed in this book.

CONTRIBUTORS

Catherine Backman, MS, OT(C), is Head, Division of Occupational Therapy, School of Rehabilitation Sciences, University of British Columbia, and is currently a doctoral candidate in Health Care & Epidemiology, also at UBC. Catherine's studies have been supported in part by the Canadian Occupational Therapy Foundation's Thelma Cardwell Scholarship. She married a stargazer and was recently sighted in a bathrobe, with binoculars aimed at Jupiter, debating how many of its moons were visible at 2 a.m.

Brian Bell was the recipient of occupational therapy services while at the Vancouver General Hospital site of VHHSC, and the G.F. Strong Rehabilitation Centre site of VHHSC. He is a strong believer in the power of the human spirit to overcome adversity and is an articulate spokesperson for client-centered practice.

Mary J. Bridle, MA, OTR/L, OT(C), FAOTA, is a Senior Occupational Therapist at the University of Virginia/HealthSouth Outpatient Therapy Service Center, Charlottesville, Virginia. During her 36-year occupational therapy career, she has been a teacher, a researcher, and a practitioner in a variety of specialty areas, including acute care, mental health, and physical rehabilitation. Besides occupational therapy, she is passionate about gardening and yoga.

Jo Clark, BSc(OT), OT(C), is the Clinical Coordinator for Occupational Therapy services at the UBCH site of Vancouver Hospital, British Columbia, Canada. She is Clinical Associate Professor in the School of Rehabilitation Sciences, University of British Columbia. She practices 1 day per week in the Ambulatory Psychiatry Clinic at UBCH and has a small private practice in the area of stress disability. Her weakness is chocolate, and her most admired public figure is the Easter Bunny.

Claire-Jehanne Dubouloz, PhD, OT(C), is an Assistant Professor in the Occupational Therapy Program at the University of Ottawa, Ontario, Canada. At present, she is pursuing two main areas of research: the development of a grounded theory of the process of transformation among diverse groups of rehabilitation clients and an exploration of evidence-based practice as a means of best practice in occupational therapy.

Mary Egan, PhD, OT(C), is an Assistant Professor in the Occupational Therapy Program at the University of Ottawa. Her research interests include the definition and promotion of evidence-based occupational therapy and the consideration of spirituality in occupational therapy practice. She dreams of singing back-up for Elvis Costello.

Virginia Griswold Fearing, BSc(OT), OT(C), OTR, is Professional Practice Director, Occupational Therapy and Music Therapy at Vancouver Hospital and Health Sciences Centre in Vancouver, British Columbia, Canada. She is Clinical Professor in the Occupational Therapy Division of the School of Rehabilitation Sciences at the University of British Columbia. She lives with a scientist and grows prize roses.

Mary Ferguson-Paré, RN, PhD, CHE, is Vice-President, Professional Affairs, Human Resources and Organizational Development at the Vancouver Hospital and Health Sciences Centre in Vancouver, Canada. She is cross-appointed to the University of British Columbia, School of Nursing, as Adjunct Professor and to the University of Victoria, School of Nursing, as Adjunct Lecturer. Her professional and academic interests include development within health care and the development of leaders who promote autonomous professional practice and a client-centered approach to service. She has a passion for the possible, a preoccupation with paradox, and a penchant for very large, lovable dogs.

Sandra Hale, BSc, OT(C), is the Section Head for Occupational Therapy services in mental health at the UBCH site of Vancouver Hospital and Health Sciences Centre and currently practices on the Mood Disorder Unit. She is a Sessional Instructor in the Occupational Therapy Program at the University of British Columbia and has a small private practice in the area of stress disability.

Mary Law, PhD, OT(C), is an Occupational Therapist with graduate training in Epidemiology and Health and Social Planning who has worked in the area of children's rehabilitation for many years. She is a Professor in the School of Rehabilitation Science and Co-Director, CanChild, Centre for Childhood Disability Research at McMaster University, Hamilton, Canada. Mary's clinical and research interests include the development, validation, and transfer into practice of outcome measures; evaluation of interventions for children with disabilities; and the study of environmental factors that affect the participation of children with disabilities. She is one of the authors of the Canadian Occupational Performance Measure, an outcome measure for occupational therapy now used in more than 30 countries around the world. She loves to go white water canoeing.

Mary Ann McColl, PhD, OT(C), is a Professor in the School of Rehabilitation Therapy at Queen's University, with a cross-appointment to the Department of Community Health and Epidemiology. She is one of the authors of the Canadian Occupational Performance Measure, as well as the author of a number of books, including *Theoretical Basis of Occupational Therapy* and *Introduction to Disability*.

Nonie Medcalf, BSc(OT), OT(C), has worked in Acute Care and Extended Care at the Vancouver Hospital & Health Sciences Centre, UBC Hospital. She is currently working as a Clinician in community health in West Vancouver, British Columbia, Canada. She wants to continue to explore the country by bicycle.

Gayle Restall, MSc, OT(C), is a Primary Health Leader for the Winnipeg Community and Long-Term Care Authority and a Sessional Instructor at the School of Medical Rehabilitation at the University of Manitoba. She has a keen interest in mental health practice spanning the life cycle from children to the elderly. Other interests include the impact of the work environment and organizational change on staff and consumers of health services and the development of accessible community health services. Gayle thrives on the peace and tranquility of Manitoba's great outdoors whether it's on a pair of cross-country skis or in a canoe.

Jacquie Ripat, MSc, OT(C), is an Instructor at the School of Medical Rehabilitation at the University of Manitoba and is the Clinical Specialist in Assistive Technology at the Health Sciences Centre in Winnipeg, Manitoba. Her current areas of interest include measuring assistive technology outcomes, validation of the Canadian Occupational Performance Measure, quantifying the effect of arthritis on an individual's kinematics and perception of disability, and facilitating client-centered approaches in a rehabilitation setting. In her quest to find the perfect leisure interest, Jacquie tries one new activity a year. Last year—curling, this year—Pilates, next year—lion taming?

Cynthia A. Stabenow, MS, OTR/L, earned a bachelor's degree from the College of Saint Catherine in St. Paul, Minnesota, in 1972 and a master's degree in Occupational Therapy from the Medical College of Virginia in 1987. In 1997, she attended a workshop on the Occupational Performance Process Model and has been using it with appropriate residents in her long-term care practice. The case study in Chapter 12 reflects her use of the Canadian Model of Occupational Performance within the constraints of the current health care delivery system in the United States.

Marlene Stern, BOT, OT(C), is the Director of Occupational Therapy, Health Sciences Centre, Winnipeg, Manitoba. She was one of the authors of the *Guidelines for Client-Centred Mental Health Practice*. Her interests include promoting client-centered environments within tertiary care facilities and expanding the roles of occupational therapists through the development of public-private partnerships. Marlene's passion for preparing fine cuisine for her family and friends is at its best when surrounded by the natural beauty of her lakeside retreat.

FOREWORD

Occupational therapy, as a profession, focuses on enabling individuals, groups, and organizations to achieve performance and satisfaction in occupations of their choice. Taking into consideration the people, their chosen occupations, and the environments in which they live, work, and play, therapists work in partnership with clients to improve occupational performance. There is considerable breadth in occupational therapists' knowledge, conceptual frameworks, practice locations, and types of individuals and groups. A significant challenge in occupational therapy practice today is to ensure that our services are client-centered, focused on occupation, and supported by research evidence. To achieve this practice goal in the midst of an ever-changing health care system, therapists require models and tools to assist them in the process, organization, and delivery of therapy services.

This book, *Individuals in Context: A Practical Guide to Client-Centered Practice* by Ginny Fearing and Jo Clark, presents the Occupational Performance Process Model (OPPM), a tool for developing a client-centered occupational therapy practice. The OPPM helps therapists to reflect and plan their service delivery to ensure that it focuses on clients' needs, is based on sound theory, is centered upon occupation, and continually evaluates the outcomes of therapy intervention. Through the use of many examples, reflective exercises, and practical tools, readers are provided with a "way to think about the occupational therapy process."

The authors of this book have had a long-standing interest in the way in which occupational therapy is provided. Guided by their commitment to the provision of client-centered, occupation-based practice, they observed and conducted studies of practice and worked with many therapists and clients to develop this model. The OPPM reflects their expertise in clinical practice and management. Student occupational therapists and practitioners will identify with the ideas put forward because they reflect real-life experience in health care today.

I have been privileged to work with Ginny and Jo as they have developed and tested the OPPM. Throughout the book, therapists are encouraged and challenged to become leaders in their profession and to put these ideas into practice. In my opinion, the use of this model on a daily basis will improve occupational therapy practice. Think of occupational therapy practice as a journey—the OPPM is your compass. It provides you with direction and the tools to reach your chosen destination. The result of this journey will be the following: an evidence-based occupational therapy practice grounded in theory and research, a client-centered practice that enhances client and therapist outcomes and satisfaction, a focus on enabling clients to perform their chosen occupations, and continual documentation of outcome and the quality of your practice.

Mary Law, PhD, OT(C)

INTRODUCTION

The purpose of this book is to provide students and therapists at any stage in their career with an opportunity to reflect on their personal practice. Through workshops on leadership and the Occupational Performance Process Model (OPPM) (Canadian Association of Occupational Therapists [CAOT], 1997; Fearing, Law, & Clark, 1997), this author has listened to hundreds of occupational therapists speak eloquently and from the heart about their clinical practice. They are eager to make client-centered practice a reality and are looking for organized ways to think about their own practice. Also, more and more clients are expressing their need to be heard and treated as individuals within the contexts of their own lives.

Individuals in Context is a response to clients, therapists, and student therapists who are seeking a way to think about the occupational therapy process. It is the result of a collaborative effort by clients and clinical and academic occupational therapists from six locations in Canada and the United States. Each chapter reflects the voices, values, and contexts of its authors, and this diversity has been intentionally preserved. As a whole, it is a multifaceted choir supporting occupational therapy students and therapists in everyday practice. As with any interesting choral piece, the reader can expect to experience a change in tempo, pace, and perhaps intensity. The themes, however, remain constant: individuals (therapists and clients alike) live within the context of their own lives and express in one way or another who they are at that moment through what they do, what they think, and how they feel.

The book begins in Section I with reflection on the congruence and relationship of leadership values to client-centered values. It continues by examining how we enable or disable through the environments we create. Section II focuses on the OPPM (CAOT, 1997; Fearing et al., 1997) with one chapter devoted to each stage of the process, one chapter illustrating a case study, and one chapter suggesting applications of the OPPM in practice. Section III addresses opportunities in a changing health care environment. The text ends with an organized approach to improve client-centered processes through self-reflection. A glossary of acronyms to assist the reader when necessary is included at the back of the book.

The OPPM, which forms the core of this book, is in no way intended to be a rigid procedure but rather a guideline for client-centered partnership and for reflection. The story that follows is a short history of the development of the OPPM. It is included here in order to encourage therapists, regardless of where they may be working, to follow their ideas, ask questions, and to risk trying new ways.

THE OPPM: A SHORT STORY

In the early 1980s, the author started puzzling over the then-current practice of therapists designing their own assessment forms. It seemed that a client-centered practice would have consistent assessments regardless of the therapist-of-the-day. If the clients' problems remained the same, shouldn't there be a systematic way to approach problem-solving?

This led to the question, "How do scientists solve problems?" Perhaps the most extraordinary part of this story is that the author ended up reading a mathematics book *How to Solve It* (Polya, 1957), a paperback book that, when purchased, had cost $0.95 U.S. and $1.10 Canadian! The basic problem-solving steps listed in Polya (1957) are:

1. Understand the problem
2. Devise a plan
3. Carry out the plan
4. Look back

At that time, of course, we did not have the Canadian Occupational Performance Measure (Law, Baptiste, Carswell, McColl, Polatajko, & Pollock, 1998) to help us "understand the problem" and "look back."

It was exciting to see that the steps occupational therapists followed to solve problems echoed the steps scientists use. It seems so simple now, and it seemed simple then. Workshops based on the four steps of problem-solving proved to be a big success with non-professional health care workers in the community. This experience heightened the author's growing awareness that a startling number of people do not problem-solve automatically or think conceptually.

In the mid-1980s, the author began to look for a systematic way to ensure continuity of client care between one therapist and another. Budget cuts had removed the then-current practice of overlapping therapists who were leaving with those who were newly hired for an orientation period as long as 2 weeks.

After some thought, it was decided that the client health record had the most potential because it was the one consistent link among therapists, team members, and the client. At that time, clients could not gain access to their health records easily, and therapists appeared to be recording in whatever way made sense to them. During workshops, the author had an opportunity to collect examples of how therapists would document client problems in the health record. For the most part, the examples were troubling, and the therapists knew it. They were definitely not satisfied with what they were doing, which is evidenced by the fact that it was not difficult at all to get 100 people to sign up for a workshop on health record documentation. Most therapists reported never having been taught how to record in a health record. Thus began years of trial and error development. Front-line staff and students have been instrumental in this development.

It seemed reasonable, because we were occupational therapists, to identify occupational performance problems, such as potential for falling in the bathroom, which we recorded on the left side of the problem list. We then recorded the components contributing to the occupational performance problems on the right side. In order to develop and implement this approach, a group of therapists from acute care, psychiatry, and extended care met regularly. Our goal was to be able to identify occupational performance problems and the components that contributed to them for each client. When we met, each therapist would bring a health record and read to the group the problem (issue) list that had been developed. When "decreased mobility" was read, we would ask, "And what does *that* look like?" We would keep asking that question until there was a description against which we could measure change, such as, "Cannot get the wheelchair through doorframes at home." There were many discussions, for example, Is sleep an occupation? Is sitting? What about breathing? And so on. Before long, and often accompanied with great hilarity, we were able to generate behavioral occupational performance statements that could be used as a baseline against which to measure progress. And further, these statements were recorded in such a way that clients could read them without discomfort. Many therapists took to this process immediately. Others were more cautious but persevered. A very few were unable to make the transition from thinking in terms of components (such as range of motion) to occupational performance.

It soon became apparent that when therapists began to think in terms of occupational performance stated in behavioral terms, they became conscious of the vague terms we were using. Anyone describing a client as being unmotivated or having low self-esteem would be met with a chorus of voices saying, "What does *that* look like?" The author is so grateful to that original group of risk-taking, open-minded therapists who discovered together the power of describing client problems in behavioral terms against which progress could be measured.

We viewed the health record as a guide for practice because plans were based on resolving occupational performance issues. It was slow going, however, as every single therapist had to be trained, or re-trained, to think in terms of occupational performance.

The author decided a visual model might assist people to "think about" the process. While playing with the idea of using both O and T, the T was superimposed on the O. Then the stem of the T was removed. While looking at what remained (an O with a line across the top), it simply came alive as the process we all go through when we lose momentum and require some assistance in problem-solving so we can regain momentum. This model depicted the "occupational therapy process as an open feedback loop through which the client may move one or more times, while learning to cope with change, until enough momentum is gathered to move into adaptation" (Fearing, 1993, p. 236).

Mary Law and Jo Clark joined this author in a collaboration, which resulted in transforming the Occupational Performance Feedback Loop into the OPPM (see Figure in *Introduction to Section II*). This transformation included organizing elements of the Feedback Loop into seven stages and adding both Stage 2, select potential intervention models, and Stage 4, identify strengths and resources. The Canadian Model of Occupational Performance (CMOP) (CAOT, 1997) graphically illustrates the dynamic relationship among person, occupation, and environment. To show the relationship of a person to the occupational performance process, the CMOP was added to the beginning of the OPPM. Before long, we had an OPPM and a paper (Fearing et al., 1997).

The OPPM was adopted with two minor changes (the word "problems" was changed to "issues" and "select potential intervention models" was changed to "select theoretical approaches") in *Enabling Occupation: An Occupational Therapy Perspective* (Stanton,

Kramer, & Thompson-Franson, 1997). The model was further explained by Fearing, Clark, and Stanton (1998) through case studies in *Client-Centered Occupational Therapy*.

While attending the 1998 World Federation of Occupational Therapists (WFOT) in Montreal, this author and Jo Clark suggested to Mary Law that we wanted to publish a manual to make the content of our workshops more accessible to therapists. Mary helped us make contact with an editor at SLACK Incorporated, and within a month we had contacted the contributing authors and had submitted a book proposal. *Individuals in Context: A Practical Guide to Client-Centered Practice* grew out of the week that we attended the WFOT conference. In this book, then, the contributing authors explore in more depth the meaning of each stage in the process. We trust that readers will make links that we have missed and will, in one way or another, move us further in the realm of infinite possibilities.

THE REALM OF INFINITE POSSIBILITIES

MacKenzie (1996) reminds us to keep our peripheral vision. He says:

> Well, in an effort to cope with the incomprehensibility of infinite reality, we ever-curious, ever-pondering, compulsively controlling Homo sapiens create theoretical models. These models are ingenious beams of speculation that we use to penetrate and define the dark mysteries of boundless existence. Sometimes elegantly structured, usually self-confirming, our models are like the headlights of a car, designed to light our way. Whatever is illuminated becomes our truth and we organize our lives around it. But this light we create can also blind us. Too often we are blinded into believing that our models are the whole reality, forgetting that they are simply useful fact/fantasy coping devices.
>
> The more fully we believe a model is reality, the more rigid the model becomes. And the more rigid it becomes, the more it confines us. There is a sense of security in this, the sense of security that comes from being contained by the "known" and thus shielded from the threat of the unknown. So the mixed blessing of models is that while they can generate a sense of coherence through a groundedness (in "knowledge"), they can also, if used without mindfulness, become addicting anesthetics to the pain of an inscrutable universe and further insulate us from full reality, which is the realm of infinite possibilities. (pp. 163-164)

The reader is challenged to take the risk of implementing the OPPM approach into practice, while remaining open to potential future development. When used as intended, this book will connect the reader with the "realm of infinite possibilities," which is the obvious result of living client-centered values and being open to learning.

Virginia (Ginny) Fearing, BSc(OT), OT(C), OTR
Vancouver, British Columbia, Canada

REFERENCES

Canadian Association of Occupational Therapists (CAOT) (1997). *Enabling occupation: An occupational therapy perspective*. Ottawa, Ontario, Canada: CAOT Publications ACE.

Fearing, V.G. (1993). Occupational therapists chart a course through the health record. *Canadian Journal of Occupational Therapy, 60,* 232-240.

Fearing, V.G., Clark, J., & Stanton, S. (1998). The client-centred occupational therapy process. In M. Law (Ed.), *Client-Centered Occupational Therapy*. Thorofare, NJ: SLACK Incorporated.

Fearing, V.G., Law, M., & Clark, J. (1997). An occupational performance process model: Fostering client and therapist alliances. *Canadian Journal of Occupational Therapy, 64,* 7-15.

Law, M., Baptiste, S., Carswell, A., McColl, M.A., Polatajko, H., & Pollock, N. (1998). *The Canadian Occupational Performance Measure (COPM)* (3rd ed.). Ottawa, Ontario, Canada: CAOT Publications.

MacKenzie, G. (1996). *Orbiting the giant hairball: A corporate fool's guide to surviving with grace*. Toronto, Ontario, Canada: Penguin Books, Ltd.

Polya, G. (1957). *How to solve it* (2nd ed.). Garden City, NY: Doubleday Anchor Books.

Stanton, S., Kramer, C., & Thompson-Franson, T. (1997). Linking concepts to a process for organizing occupational therapy services. In Canadian Association of Occupational Therapists, *Enabling Occupation: An Occupational Therapy Perspective*. Ottawa, Ontario, Canada: CAOT Publications.

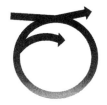

REFLECTING ON THERAPISTS IN CONTEXT

chapter one

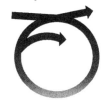

LEADERSHIP IN DAILY PRACTICE

VIRGINIA G. FEARING, BSc(OT), OT(C), OTR,
MARY FERGUSON-PARÉ, RN, PHD, CHE

This chapter is about who you are as an individual and what you bring to the client-therapist partnership. The framework used for this introspection will be based in leadership literature. Chapter 2, *Environments that Enable Therapist and Client Occupations*, further explores the client-therapist partnership and the shared environment that is created.

What does leadership have to do with occupational therapy practice? Because both leadership and client-centered practice are driven by values, therapists will benefit from reflecting on their personal view of what leadership "looks like" and how it is similar to, or different from, the way they practice. Leadership and client-centered practice are frequently used words that mean different things to different people. That is because our personal view of leadership and client-centered practice reflects our own values and the mental models that we hold at the time. Understanding that deeply felt values are generally the source of both leadership and client-centered behaviors alerts us to the need to reflect on our own values in order to understand not only what drives our personal leadership but also our professional practice.

If each of us identified five nationally or internationally known people who we believed exemplified leadership, would we agree on either the people selected or our reasons for selecting them? Would we agree on which leadership behaviors caught our attention? Another way to think about what leadership "looks like" is to identify five people who are providing leadership in the context of your own life. What behaviors did you use as criteria for selection?

Does leadership mean that there are those who follow? It is important to examine the behaviors not only of those who lead but also of those who are led in order to appreciate the values conveyed in leadership. For example, thousands of people demonstrated strength and courage through non-violent behavior because of Mahatma Gandhi's leadership. This tells us something about how Mahatma Gandhi's values resonated with others. Would he still be considered a leader if others had not followed? Consider the people you identified as leaders in the context of your own life. What behaviors do you exhibit as a result of their leadership? Are those leaders aware that they have influenced you?

You may discover that the leadership you value reflects the "leader-as-enabler" more than the "leader-of-those-who-follow." It was Gandhi who said, "The leader is not the person with the most followers: the leader is the one who creates the most leaders." This chapter addresses leadership in a client-therapist process and then leadership within the context of organizations.

LEADERSHIP THAT ENABLES

"Leaders who learn from, teach, serve, and empower others—particularly their customers, clients, and others—are tomorrow" (Batten, 1998, p. 39). Today, occupational therapists pride themselves in enabling others, often without understanding that enabling **is** leadership. "One of the most persistent myths in our culture associates leadership with rank. But leadership isn't a position; it's a process" (Kouzes, 1998, p. 322). Leadership for the future is not about controlling from a position of power, but about enabling from a position in partnership. An enabling style of leadership springs from a way of being-with-others that permeates every interaction. Chapters 3 through 9 use the Occupational Performance Process Model (Fearing, Law, & Clark, 1997) to guide therapists through a way of being-with-others that reflects both client-centered values and leadership that enables.

Bender (1997) teaches that we are moving toward a new definition of leadership that "begins with leading **ourselves**" (p. 5). He argues that "powerful leadership comes from knowing yourself" (p. xiv). The importance of self-reflection regarding personal values, beliefs, and principles cannot be overemphasized. We must ask ourselves, "Who am I?" "What do I stand for?" The reason for this is that we are structuring and co-creating meaning in everything we do, and this meaning varies based on perceptions, values, and sociocultural context. "Are my values truly about partnership with clients?" "Do I really believe in practice centered around the client?" Whether or not we are aware of them, we literally express our values, beliefs, and principles in everything we do and in all of the approaches we choose in each relationship within the practice environment.

Occupational therapy values and beliefs, as identified in *Enabling Occupation: An Occupational Therapy Perspective* (Canadian Association of Occupational Therapists [CAOT], 1997), form a basis for reflection on professional values for occupational therapists. Do we agree with each value, and, if so, which of our behaviors might other people recognize as living those values? Believing that "client-centered practice in occupational therapy focuses on enabling occupation" (CAOT, 1997, p. 31) will result in identifiable behaviors. A dissonance between what we **say** we value and what we **do** is obvious to others and is worthy of reflection. Because client-centered practice is all about human relationships, it is important to know ourselves and to appreciate the differences among us.

In general, we all have a personal way of managing our lives, our relationships, and the challenges that face us. Contrary to what we may sometimes experience, that uniqueness is precious and to be honored for its expression of individual humanity and for its contribution to a society enriched by diversity and by acceptance. Regardless of other people's opinions, the methods we use to manage our daily lives are generally effective, although often unique and sometimes remarkable. Periodically, however, a person or group of people will choose to learn a different way of doing things, or perhaps will be forced to alter long-held habits and patterns due to trauma or illness of one kind or another. Whatever the cause, whether as a result of choice or circumstances, people may find themselves in a client-therapist process. This process requires leadership from both the client and therapist.

CLIENT AS LEADER

As master of a personal journey in life, individual clients and their families are recognized as experts in context, in values, in personal hopes, and in dreams. Moreover, these change, requiring the therapist to be in tune with where that individual is in the process of living. Clients enable the therapeutic process by being themselves, by making choices that resonate with their own values, and by teaching us. Clients or families labeled as "difficult" or "demanding" are often trying to assume leadership for their own situation, making a bold and clear statement in the way they know best. Although this is a good sign, it can be threatening to therapists who miss the meaning behind the behavior. What the therapist may perceive as a threat to the way-we-do-things (and it probably is) may be seen from the client's perspective as an expression of self-determination. "This works for me." "We do not agree with your recommendations." "I always do it this way." "I need to know what is going on." These are examples of meanings and values that are all too often misunderstood. The meaning clients give to change and to the client-therapist partnership is important and can influence their self-perception, their confidence in personal choice, and their will to continue.

When clients are recognized as leaders in a client-centered process, they are free to think about and communicate a personal vision for their future and to make the choices that will get them there. They can set goals relevant to their own future and expect support and assistance from the therapist to achieve them. They will use partnerships to extend their skills and abilities, and they will change their partner when the fit is poor. This clearly means that the therapist's work with a client must be based on valuing the client's choices in that partnership. The concept of client as leader-partner is very different from the traditional expectation that the therapist controls, knows best, and keeps a professional distance from the client. The quest for client-centered practice reflects the struggle we have had in being unsure of who we are and therefore needing to be seen as expert and in control while at the same time considering ourselves client-centered.

THERAPIST AS LEADER

Self-knowledge forms the stable base from which therapists can find comfort with both following and leading, attending to self and to client, learning and teaching, being expert and being novice, and working toward a valued future while attending to the present process. Opening a space for client-centered process is an important part of leadership in occupational therapy daily practice. This means deliberately creating an interpersonal environment in which the values inherent in client-centered practice can be expressed and in which clients themselves can live those values in determining and charting their goals and life plans. This is not as easy to do as it sounds. In order to bring client-centered values alive every day, occupational therapists must have a deep understanding and respect for the fact that we are all masters of our own journey in life. We all express ourselves through how we live our lives, the choices we make, the stories we tell, and the contexts we live within.

As a result of giving expression to who we are within the context of our own lives, we are continually changing and learning about ourselves. Who the client is and who the therapist is changes constantly. "No one can judge another person's process, and frequently we cannot even understand it" (Schaef, 1998, p. 237). We can only seek to understand and to provide needed support. Perhaps the biggest challenge in all relationships, personal or therapeutic, is learning to provide support and making room for unexpected choices as the individual searches for and finds meaning from within. Anyone who has listened to someone else tell them what to do, while silently thinking it might be good advice **but** would never work in **this** particular situation, will understand.

Clearly, part of therapist leadership is creating a space for valuing client leadership. This means being comfortable with the variety of ways in which people express who they are and being open to learning from them. When the client is valued as expert-in-context, therapists continuously learn and experience comfort being novice-in-context while in no way being threatened about areas of expertise. One of the hardest lessons therapists learn is how to provide leadership while following where the client leads. Therapists who find themselves labeling clients as "difficult," "non-compliant," "demanding," or "not motivated" will benefit from reflecting on whether or not there has been space created for client leadership.

Another hard lesson is to recognize client behavior that is part of processing life's events, without labeling the client as "not coping" or "unmotivated." Laughter, tears, and all expression of feelings are part of living the current process as well as incorporating it into a meaningful memory for the future. "...for the leader with self-knowledge, emotion is not a dangerous spark to be smothered; rather it is an ember from which other activities gain warmth, energy, and meaning" (O'Neil, 1997, p. 115). Therapists who are aware of their own expression of humanity and its impact on others are able to stand beside clients in a non-controlling, non-judgmental way, as clients discover a future they can live and work for, within the context of their own lives. Therapist leadership, then, is based on a foundation of understanding self, believing in self and client, and bringing healthy approaches to practice.

ORGANIZATIONS AS CONTEXT FOR LEADERSHIP IN DAILY PRACTICE

Readers may be wondering how to make a space for client-centered practice within their current practice environment, whatever that may be. As therapists, we have a commitment to the client to ensure that the client-therapist process is focused on addressing client issues. In addition, we have a commitment to the employer. Organizations have a dual commitment as well, to the clients and to the staff whose expertise and attitude are critical to client-centered practice. Organizations are nothing more than large families of people. By the nature of their size, organizations create a complexity that requires clarification of collective values and purpose for being. Remembering that **we are** the organization assists us in finding the courage to act from an enabling, or leadership, position. Thinking of leadership on a continuum, rather than in a hierarchy, makes it possible to see how leadership behaviors can be applied on an individual, group, corporate, national, or international level. Covey (1998, p. xvii) paraphrases Senge (1990a, p. 64), who drew upon Buckminster Fuller's description of leverage, "A trim tab is the small rudder that moves the big rudder that moves the whole ship. If a person can become the trim tab, he or she can move an entire organization."

Management may or may not be synonymous with leadership. Even when it is, "Organizations today cannot survive if leadership is limited to the CEOs, executives, and managers" (Bergmann, Hurson, & Russ-Eft, 1999, p.16). From their studies, Bergmann et al. have identified a grassroots model of leadership that is not role dependent. They report that grassroots leaders "help others personalize a future for themselves," "navigate through emotional ups and downs," are "not afraid of midcourse adjustments," and "find a way to maintain a sense of optimism" (p. 23). When we choose to practice from a client-centered position, we are choosing, among other things, to take responsibility for using ourselves to make room for others to be not only who they are now but also who they choose to become.

It can be very lonely to live our leadership and client-centered values. It helps to believe in the power of a single voice. When one person hums a tune that connects to the values of others, it will resonate and can lead to others joining in and eventually to a whole choir of voices. Of course, if the person humming the tune is discordant or abrasive, there is the risk of being avoided, or worse. There is always that risk if the tune is new and does not fit the expectations or values of others. However, for the person singing, the melody and the message remain. One therapist, who chooses to practice from a client-centered position in an environment where client-centered process is not recognizable, can start by humming the client-centered tune. This may be more effective than trying to get together a choir of unbelievers and expecting harmony. Hum the tune that expresses your values and satisfaction with the way you practice, and watch what happens around you over time. In the words of Nelson Mandela, "There's nothing enlightened about shrinking so that other people won't feel insecure around you…As we let our own light shine, we unconsciously give other people permission to do the same" (O'Neil, 1997, p. 174).

Where either the organizational or practice environments are not supportive, the leadership rests with the therapist and client to create, in partnership, an enabling environment relevant to the client's and therapist's mutual work. Therapists and clients are challenged to move out of the victim role and take responsibility for their shared leadership even when the environment of the organization is not enabling. The authors can say from personal experience that on a human level it is very difficult to carry on in a hostile environment but it can be done. It challenges values and sense of self and creates a readiness to leave and seek alternatives. This is a natural response to being in an environment not congruent with our values. It is important to reflect on the source of the feeling of disconnect. Having acknowledged that, we can go forward humming our tune. This may become the point where fight or flight occurs. However, one of the greatest sources of job satisfaction for therapists comes from what we can do together with clients. It is possible to find personal satisfaction by focusing on what is important within the organization without being sucked into the organizational "hairball," as charmingly portrayed by MacKenzie (1996) in *Orbiting the Giant Hairball.*

Organizations typically convey expectations about the nature of leadership within the organization through structuring elements such as the vision, values, and mission statements. Ideally, these statements support client-centered practice. Clear communication through these stated expectations about a client-centered approach to service, teaching, and research contributes to making a space for client-centered practice. Then, expectations for practice are demonstrated through role modeling within the environment. Ultimately, this vision needs to be jointly held. It is known that high performing organizations work together with staff at all levels to create a mutual vision for the organization and then engage in activities to communicate this throughout the organization to influence practice. It is best if organizations are bold and clear about all activities relating to the vision, values, and mission of the organization. Wilma Mankiller, former Chief of the Cherokee nation, was described as "the best kind of leader: one who creates independence, not dependence" (Steinem, 1992, p. 98). A leadership style that supports client-centered practice is based in empowerment. When a corporation chooses to support client-centered practice through its vision and values, it can be a very powerful support to therapists seeking to practice in this way.

The expectations that organizations convey through their vision, values, and mission statements may be different from what is **enacted** through corporate decision-making and through generally accepted practice. Understanding the corporate context involves monitoring not only what the organization says but also what it does. Whether we are an individual or a corporation, saying we are client-centered does not make us so. The first step, however, is having a vision of what client-centered practice looks like. The second step is to build a shared vision with others.

Organizations generally designate formal leaders whose values may or may not resonate with client-centered practice. Leaders successful in promoting empowerment in practice in a team-based environment have a particular human quality. They provide the necessary structures to ensure quality and standards and provide policy direction and individual direction to practitioners where needed. But they do so in a supportive manner that focuses on recognizing and building on the strengths and commitments of practitioners through the mutual development of vision and the support of life-long learning to build the team in which they work. These leaders also support direct empowerment of practitioners through continuous development and sharing responsibility for decision-making.

Ferguson-Paré (1998) conducted a study of managers that revealed that consideration behaviors are also empowering management behaviors. In the leadership literature, consideration behaviors are the supportive human behaviors of the leader. They are built around an approachable, friendly relationship with practitioners where the manager listens, provides direct recognition for good work, and supports and advocates for practitioners while regarding them as competent team players. These managers are constantly upgrading their education and developing themselves to better support and develop practitioners and teams. They use cooperative approaches to problem-solving in which they collaborate with practitioners, each contributing unique expertise toward a common end. They demonstrate a very positive view of staff as competent, independent practitioners at various levels of development. Use of vision and a holistic approach to people through the demonstration of personal interest in staff, addressing the spiritual or psychosocial aspects of people, and the use of appropriate touch are critical attributes of these managers. The development of managers who exhibit these human, professional, and leadership qualities will contribute to the supports necessary to empower practitioners. Quality of work life for therapists and quality of client-centered practice are inseparable and bound in the same value structure.

In reality, the relationship therapists experience with managers may not fit this description. Then the therapist must create a personal context, reviewing how to use self to address issues, remaining focused on what is important, and remaining true to personal values. It is important to give voice to needs and what is valued in order to carry out client-centered practice and to build a choir within the team.

DEVELOPING CONGRUENCE BETWEEN VALUES AND BEHAVIORS

Reflecting on the fit of our personal values with client-centered and leadership values, and the dissonance between what we believe and what we do, can lead to painful self-discovery. Regardless of comfort level, this process of self-discovery is critical to effective practice. Every reflective therapist must make serious choices. Shall I invest the time and energy it takes to engage in the life-long learning required for client-centered practice, or shall I self-select out of this profession? If I choose to remain in the profession, what will my commitment to learning look like? Leaders in organizations that value learning are responsible for building organizations where people are continually expanding their capabilities to shape their future, that is, leaders are responsible for learning (Senge, 1990b).

Because we are continually learning and changing, reflection is an ongoing part of any vital practice. This reflection can help focus our energies for the future. Fearing and Clark

(1998) use a simple method to guide therapists through interactive or personal reflection on how they practice. It also serves as a map for continued development.

This is how it works:

1. Make a list of 8 to 12 behaviors that exemplify client-centered practice.
2. Then make a list of 8 to 12 behaviors that exemplify leadership. It may help to visualize people you know personally. Name their valued behaviors.
3. Compare the lists, and consider the similarities and the differences.
4. From this total list, select the 12 behaviors you value most highly, and place one at the tip of each star point in Figure 1-1. Place those behaviors that you value highly on the longest points.
5. Compare what you value (placed on the star points) with how you behave. Start in the center of the star. If you think you are in great shape physically, mentally, and functionally, you will simply draw on top of the circle represented by a dotted line. If you are feeling out of shape physically, draw that part of the circle closer to the center. Now assess mental and functional health in the same way. This center circle is the self that forms the healthy basis from which leadership and client-centered behaviors are expressed. On reflection, you may see that you are in no shape to support the star points and therefore probably are unable to invest energy in leadership or client-centered behaviors. A healthy self comes first.
6. Now, consider each star point item. Thinking of the center of the star as "not at all" and the tip of the star as "personal strengths and integrated into the way I practice," place an "o" along the continuum from star point to star center that best describes your usual behaviors. This will be different for each person and for each star point. Once you have completed this reflection for each item, draw a new star, connecting the points you have drawn, creating a new star that is your personal map. Figure 1-2 is an example of a partially completed Leadership Star.
7. Choose two behaviors that are important to your effective practice and that you would like to change.
8. For each behavior you have selected, identify two people you know who exemplify excellence in that area.
9. Contact these people. Negotiate their coaching assistance as you learn behaviors in which they excel. Our experience is that this type of mentoring often turns into mutual support for ongoing leadership development.
10. Ask a colleague to fill out the leadership star as he or she perceives you, and then compare it with your own. Share the differences and similarities with your colleague.
11. Review your personal leadership star regularly. This provides you with an opportunity to acknowledge your accomplishments and to plan for the next ones.

One of the authors has chosen two behaviors to develop: the use of healthy humor especially in tense situations and the ability to focus on listening. Selecting people who exemplified those behaviors was easy. Approaching them to seek coaching took courage but resulted in thoughtful and sometimes surprising discussions. The greatest benefits have been an increased awareness and the commitment to learn specific behaviors.

Leaders in everyday occupational therapy practice hum a tune that resonates with clients. They hum a tune that reflects client-centered values. They are a joy to work with because they respect every human being. This chapter set out to provoke a dialogue within yourself that has the potential to lead you to a stronger place in your own practice and to create a stronger workplace by your example. "You must be the change you wish to see in the world" (Gandhi).

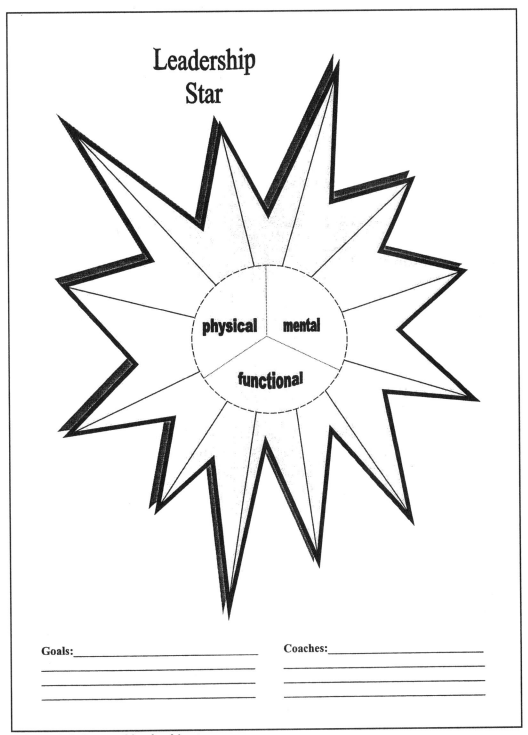

Figure 1-1. Personal leadership star.

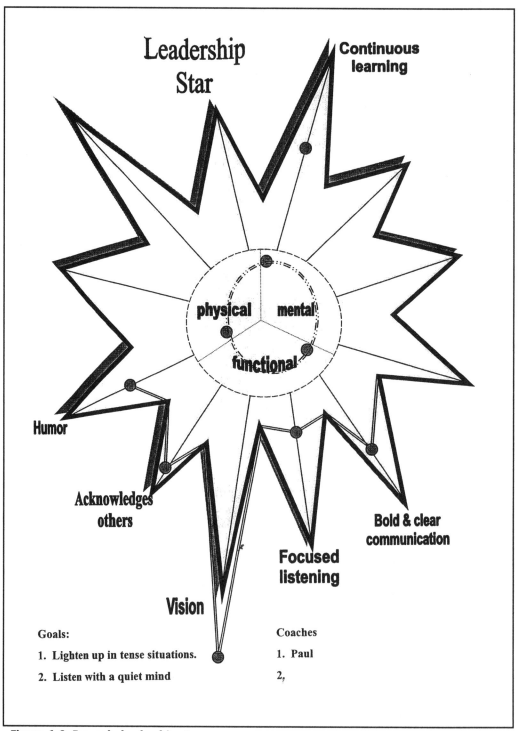

Figure 1-2. Example leadership star.

REFERENCES

Batten, J. (1998). Servant-leadership: A passion to serve. In L.C. Spears (Ed.), *Insights on Leadership: Service, Stewardship, Spirit, and Servant-Leadership*. Toronto, Ontario, Canada: John Wiley & Sons, Inc.

Bender, P.U. (with Hellman, E.) (1997). *Leadership from within*. Toronto, Ontario, Canada: Stoddart Publishing Co. Ltd.

Bergmann, H., Hurson, K., & Russ-Eft, D. (1999). *Everyone a leader: A grassroots model for the new workplace*. New York: John Wiley & Sons, Inc.

Canadian Association of Occupational Therapists (CAOT) (1997). *Enabling occupation: An occupational therapy perspective*. Ottawa, Ontario, Canada: CAOT Publications ACE.

Covey, S.R. (1998). Foreword. In L.C. Spears (Ed.), *Insights on Leadership: Service, Stewardship, Spirit, and Servant-Leadership*. Toronto, Ontario, Canada: John Wiley & Sons, Inc.

Fearing, V.G., & Clark, J. (1998). *Reflecting on personal leadership behaviors*. Unpublished raw data.

Fearing, V.G., Law, M., & Clark, J. (1997). An occupational performance process model: Fostering client and therapist alliances. *Canadian Journal of Occupational Therapy, 64*, 7-15.

Ferguson-Paré, M. (1998). Nursing leadership and autonomous professional practice of registered nurses. *Canadian Journal of Nursing Administration, 11*(2), 7-30.

Kouzes, J.M. (1998). Finding your voice. In L.C. Spears (Ed.), *Insights on Leadership: Service, Stewardship, Spirit, and Servant-Leadership*. Toronto, Ontario, Canada: John Wiley & Sons, Inc.

MacKenzie, G. (1996). *Orbiting the giant hairball: A corporate fool's guide to surviving with grace*. Toronto, Ontario, Canada: Penguin Books Ltd.

O'Neil, J. (1997). *Leadership Aikido: 6 business practices to turn around your life*. New York: Harmony Books.

Schaef, A.W. (1998). *Living in process: Basic truths for living the path of the soul*. Toronto, Ontario, Canada: Random House.

Senge, P.M. (1990a). *The fifth discipline: The art and practice of the learning organization* (pp. 64-65). New York: Doubleday.

Senge, P.M. (1990b). The leader's new work: Building learning organizations. *Sloane Management Review, 32*(1), 9.

Steinem, G. (1992). *Revolution from within: A book of self-esteem*. Toronto, Ontario, Canada: Little, Brown & Co.

chapter two

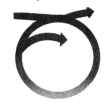

Environments that Enable Therapist and Client Occupations

Virginia G. Fearing, BSc(OT), OT(C), OTR

This chapter focuses on how we can use ourselves to co-create healthy and enabling environments with clients through our presence, our communication, and our presentation.

Occupational therapists believe that "environment is a broad term including cultural, institutional, physical, and social components" and that "performance, organization, choice, and satisfaction in occupations are determined by the relationship between persons and their environment" (Canadian Association of Occupational Therapists, 1997, p. 31); that is, that there is an interdependence among people, their environments, and their occupations (Law, Cooper, Strong, Stewart, Rigby, & Letts, 1996; Strong, Rigby, Stewart, Law, Letts, & Cooper, 1999). This reminds us that the connections that clients make in the client-therapist environment are critical to their performance, their choices, and their satisfaction.

Occupational therapy is an interactive process, requiring knowledge of many therapeutic techniques and interventions and great skill in the art of connecting with an infinite variety of human beings who are simply trying to live their lives in ways that have meaning for them. "As human beings we have to acknowledge that we do not exist in isolation. Unfortunately, we so easily forget that we exist in context and that there is no way to understand ourselves in isolation. We are connectedness. We are unique. And we exist in context" (Schaef, 1998, p. 228).

One way to think about personal context is to visualize an imaginary hub around each individual that carries the present manifestation of all that has gone before. This personal hub will reflect, among other things, belief in self, joys, pain, worries, or distractions of any kind through a variety of behaviors that have meaning in that person's context. The meaning of these behaviors may not be immediately obvious to others and can trigger reactions that get in the way of a healthy client-therapist process. It is important to note that both the therapist and the client carry personal hubs. These hubs differ from day to day, from hour to hour, and from person to person. The way these personal contexts (hubs) interface with each other is critical to enabling environments.

In enabling environments, people feel safe to be themselves, to do what matters to them, to become the people they want to be, and to interact with others in healthy ways that have meaning. In order for us to co-create enabling environments with clients, we heighten our awareness of what we bring to that environment and are prepared to alter our interaction style and approaches so that we contribute health to the client-therapist context.

Often when thinking of enabling environments, we focus on physical environment. Is the space accessible? Does it protect client confidentiality? Are the chairs comfortable and at a useful height? Is the room temperature comfortable? These are important questions to ask regarding environments, and occupational therapists generally excel at these questions and answers. The greater challenge, however, is to consider how we enable others, and ourselves, through the way we choose to be present, how we communicate, and the way we present ourselves.

PRESENCE

Presence refers to the degree to which we are totally present in the client-therapist process. It can be wonderfully validating to have the complete presence of another person.

> *It is easy to choose not to be present: We may drift off in our thoughts, be emotionally embroiled in a past problem, or be dreaming about future possibilities. In this case it can be truly said that we're "not all there." You have probably experienced the absence of someone who was present. We do it to others all of the time. When we choose to "show up" energetically, with all four intelligences [**mental**, **emotional**, **spiritual**, and **physical**], we express the power of presence.* (Arrien, 1993, p. 23)

Mental presence requires a quiet mind, one that is not busy thinking about what to have for supper, the work left to do, or what to say next. Mental presence is focused on this moment, not on the past or the future. This focused attention is required for deep listening. Profound listening occurs when we concentrate and when we notice what is happening in the moment (Goldstein, 1976). Shaeffer (1996) tells us that there is a difference between active listening and deep listening. "The difference is subtle yet profound. In active listening I continue to act as if words are objects." In active listening, it is important to hear the other person correctly and so we check it out. For example, "What I hear you say is…" In deep listening, knowing that it is impossible to truly understand another person's words, "…we listen to ourselves, to the meaning we experience within as we hear the words of others." We learn to sense and to express the meanings raised by the speaker's words and to seek similarities between the listener's and the speaker's meanings. "The feeling I sense within [myself] as I hear your words is…" (p. 41). In this way, we check out, not the words, but the feeling and meaning behind the words. This is an art and can lead to people feeling listened to for the first time.

We are lucky if listeners are focused on understanding the meaning of our words rather than finishing our sentences, interrupting, interpreting, moving on. The act of speaking our thoughts out loud gives us the opportunity to listen to ourselves and can be pivotal to working through what we need to do next. It is difficult to think through what we need to do when someone else assumes he or she knows what we are going to say and continually prompts us. Keeping a mind that is quiet enough to really be with self and with another person is an act of will. It is not easy to do and requires conscious attention.

The dialogue that follows deep listening is at an altogether different level than the dialogue that occurs when we exchange thoughts without connecting at the level of meaning. Consider, for example, a scenario where as a client you tell the therapist you are angry and he responds, in active listener mode, by saying, "What I hear you say is that you are angry." In this case, you would confirm that you are angry. Alternatively, consider a scenario where you tell the same person you are angry and he responds in deep listener mode: "As I hear your words and watch your actions, it reminds me of an anger I have had that feels helpless. Does that have meaning for you?" In this second scenario, you, as client, would likely begin to explore the quality of anger and its meaning in your life. If the listener missed the mark, and this does happen, you might reply that you do not feel helpless at all but ready to do damage. This can lead to further discussion and clarification of meaning. When the listener is able to match meaning, the speaker feels heard and can begin to move on. The active listener reflects the mood. The deep listener validates, looks for conjoint feelings, and explores meaning. The advisor listener, a very easy mode to fall into, simply tells the client how to respond, for example, "You tell her to get lost." The active listener, the deep listener, and the advisor listener elicit different responses.

What cues do you get from other people that convince you that they understand the meaning of your words? How often are you able to deeply listen to others? Some of us will spend a lifetime learning to be deep listeners, to ask questions rather than give answers, and to be comfortable with silence in the room and in our own minds.

Physical presence is the outward manifestation of attention. When our attention is scattered, our physical presence will convey that. Alternatively, when our attention is focused, our physical presence will convey that, too. What outward cues might others pick up during conversation with you that indicate your attention, or lack of it? Consider where you position yourself in relation to the other. Consider eye contact. What are you doing with your hands? How often do you interrupt and, more importantly, why? Are you interrupting to clarify meaning or to answer the telephone?

What physical cues do you get from others that they are present with, or absent from, you? Sensitivity to physical presence can lead to useful information. Perhaps the way you are conveying information is boring or sailing right over the head of the listener, who responds by fidgeting or exhibiting other behaviors that convey the need to depart. Perhaps the meaning of the fidgeting is pain. It could be lack of time. To co-create an enabling client-therapist environment, it is important to question what needs to be done to enable physical presence of the client and of the therapist.

Spiritual presence requires suspension of judgment. Openness and acceptance, characteristics of spiritual presence, are calming and promote connections. Spiritual presence conveys to self and others that we are what we are, we are in this world together, and we are whole. Developing spiritual presence is a deeply personal journey. This author believes it involves knowing and accepting self so that personal issues are not played out through others. It involves bringing empathy and compassion with our presence. Rather than picking up and carrying the issues of others, we transform them by understanding, validating, believing, and, at our deepest core, wishing people well. The stability, hope, and open-mindedness that are embedded in spiritual presence contribute to the sense of a safe place from which to leap into the future.

Emotional presence requires an acceptance and comfort with self that precludes the need to be the center of attention, to control, to be "right." Part of emotional presence is sensitivity to emotional boundaries, recognizing what emotions belong to whom. The therapist who is not defending self or talking other people out of their feelings is in a position to facilitate a process that incorporates validation, ventilation, and resolution.

Emotional presence includes listening for and validating meanings, and holding space for clients to acknowledge and express their feelings. Ross, in *The Fifth Discipline Fieldbook* (1994), speaks of the "ladder of inference" we climb when we start with observable data and, through inference, end with actions based on our beliefs. The first rung of the ladder is observable data, and then, within our minds, we climb the inference rungs of selecting certain data, adding meanings, making assumptions, and then drawing conclusions on which to form beliefs that then translate into action. In order to have fewer self-generated beliefs based on our assumptions, we become more aware of our own thinking and reasoning (reflection), make our own thinking and reasoning more visible to others (advocacy), and inquire into others' thinking and reasoning (inquiry).

One indicator of emotional presence is the ability to laugh with and at self in a healthy way. In *Humor and the Health Professions* (2nd ed.) (Robinson, 1991), we are reminded that humor is a familiar and informal form of communication. This informative book leads the reader through different styles and uses of humor. Humor functions on a continuum from "simple nonsense, pleasure to warmth, to social need, to anxieties, to anger, and to the deeper psychological needs around tragedy and death" (p. 46). Robinson admonishes us to listen to the joking by clients, which will reveal their latest (perhaps latent) anxieties and fears.

Not long ago, the author was with a group of a dozen occupational therapists who have worked together for a long time. It soon became apparent that they laughed often, and also that they attended to the laughter, looking at each other and just appreciating the moment. There was an "isn't it great to be alive" quality to their laughter—healing laughter. On the other hand, we have probably all known at least one person who hides behind humor. It is also worth remembering that laughter can be cruel and act as a barrier to healthy communication. Is humor part of your environment? Would others describe your style of humor as healthy?

A major barrier to being physically, mentally, spiritually, and emotionally present in the moment and in the conversation is the pressure we allow ourselves to experience as "too much work" to do. Whyte (1994) reminds us that "The rich flow of creativity, innovation, and almost musical complexity we are looking for in a fulfilled work life cannot be reached through trying or working harder." He goes on to speak of "an ever-moving first-hand creative engagement with life and with others that completes itself simply by *being* itself" (p. 298). Being in the moment requires presence. Being present makes it possible to listen to others, and also to self. It was Gandhi who taught us that there is more to life than increasing its speed.

Some of us work in environments where it is considered the norm to be stressed. To demonstrate our value, we race around wailing our stress to all those who will listen. We answer phones in the middle of conversations. We arrive late and with fanfare at meetings, explaining to all that we are just swamped. We send spoken and unspoken messages that we are too busy for interactions that have meaning. We just generally look disorganized.

> *When a corporation prizes those who are heroically overworked in stress-filled jobs,*
> *a siren song whispers to everyone else in the organization:*
> *Make your job difficult,*
> *stretch yourself thin,*
> *stress yourself out and eventually you, too,*
> *may be honored with executive approval.* (MacKenzie, 1996, p. 59)

Creating an enabling environment requires that therapists attend to their own health in such a way that they can be fully present with clients. Attending to personal health means being aware of and managing our own internal and external workload, homeload, and playload in such a way that it no longer feels like a load. Making space for client-centered practice and then filling that space with therapist stress is counter-productive.

It is long past time for us to stop and think about how the "I'm stressed" method of coping insulates us from having to be truly present with anyone. How can we be present when we are rushing into the future? The self-inflicted expectation that we will spend all our time "doing" and no time "reflecting" is a barrier to practice and puzzling among professionals who speak of balance in life. "Moving toward stillness means taking time out from the 'real' work to focus inwardly. For leaders it means carving time out of the schedule for people to reflect on what they truly want their work to be about" (Klein & Izzo, 1999, p. 76). Sometimes, because of our personal contexts, the person we may be in that moment is tired. A balance of activity and reflection not only allows us to listen, but creates a buffer that gives us the energy to be who we are in that moment. MacKenzie (1996) suggests that we "make room in our minds for the possibility that, sometimes, when [we] see a colleague whose job seems easy, [we] may in fact be witnessing a champion at play" (p. 59). We exemplify our commitment to a balanced lifestyle and to health by the way we live our lives.

A balanced approach to practice that makes it possible to be present with others can be approached through different avenues. Here are three. The first is to take responsibility for organizing how time will be spent, setting boundaries to what it is possible and reasonable to do, and building in time for reflection. "...We must learn to balance ourselves between urgency and stillness....Too much urgency turns our efforts compulsive; we are active but not productive" (Klein & Izzo, 1999, p. 197). Creating an environment balanced with doing and reflecting enhances both. Organizing time is a continuous process that requires reflection on what is important. Once our priorities are clear, we more clearly communicate to others what they can expect from us.

The second approach is to increase awareness and reflect on how our presence influences the environment. Recognizing that it is not possible to achieve 100% of our expectations at all times, through reflection, we can learn to recognize warning signs within others and within ourselves that they or we are absent mentally, physically, spiritually, or emotionally. These red alerts remind us to clarify meanings, especially in relation to what is important to the client. We may learn that our promptness is critical to their trust in us. Or that privacy is critical. Or that we have not matched our pace to theirs. Or that we are overwhelmed. Whatever we learn, it should move us beyond the presence that is absent.

The third approach is to create with others a learning environment that values and promotes moving beyond what we know.

> *We are limited by what we know. Paradoxically, we are limited by the very knowledge that has been the basis of our past success. Knowledge, which by definition is related to the past, cannot help us create the future. As long as we rely on the knowledge and answers of our past, we will be compelled to perpetuate the past.* (Klein & Izzo, 1999, p. 177)

A true learning environment promotes presence, just as presence promotes learning. Understanding the meaning in the lives of other people requires continuous learning. The therapist who role models continuous learning and comfort with being a continuous novice contributes to an environment that values growing, changing, and diversity of opinion. Comfort with being a novice means that we can be present in the give and take, the openness, and the thrill of discovery that accompanies learning. The quality of learning environment we are seeking ensures that both the therapist and client can be "awestruck with wonder, ripe with the dumbest questions, and thirsting to learn" (Whyte, 1994, p. 290). When we create true learning environments, we become open to infinite possibilities, willing to set aside plans and follow where the learner leads. Because occupational therapy is all about learning and assisting others to learn, it is curious that there has not been a greater focus on understanding and creating learning environments.

COMMUNICATION

Whether intended or not, the way we choose to be present is received as communication by the other person. We communicate through what we say, what we do, and how we listen. Making assumptions from behaviors without checking those assumptions out is both common and very dangerous. It can lead to great misunderstanding. If I am distracted with worry about my sick child at home, and you assume or read into my abrupt behaviors that I do not care what happens to you, missed communication has occurred.

It is important to carefully consider the difference between truth telling and complaining. As therapists, we ask people to talk to us about their issues. Many people experience discomfort with this because they do not want to be perceived as complaining. They want to please us and so edit their stories. We can make people more comfortable telling their stories when we understand and explain to them that truth telling often leads to action, whether it is overt action or increased understanding. Complaining tends to reoccur without resulting in action. Therapists who hear truth telling as complaining are missing a vital communication link.

The author who had known she was deaf in one ear for years was shocked to find herself devastated by a physician who said to her as he passed her in the waiting room following an exam, "Yep, you have a dead ear." It took 2 days to sort out the meaning of the unexpected but very real emotional reaction. Although not hearing, the ear was very much alive—warm to the touch, connected to the body, and part of a whole presentation. Had the physician bothered to ask about the meaning of this ear in the context of a whole life, he would have learned that in a whimsical sort of way this ear, though deaf, had long been considered the one that listens within, rather than without. The message, "dead ear," was delivered in passing in the context of a crowded waiting room. There is a big difference between deaf and dead.

"Communication that carries integrity always considers timing and context before the delivery of content" (Arrien, 1993, p. 83). Therapists committed to creating enabling environments consider the time, the place, and the content before communicating. This makes it possible not only to be heard but also to connect with the response of the person listening. Communication is often thought of as speaking, but a vital part of communication is listening. Many of us know people who drop verbal bombs as they walk out the door, leaving the listener reeling with reaction. "Skillful communication means we have aligned content, timing, and context. Blunt communication is an announcement of great content, but poor timing and context. Confused communication often carries good timing and context but poor content, and leads to incongruity between our words and our behavior" (Arrien, 1993, p. 24). If we believe that trust is based on congruity between words and actions, then the relationships between what we say and what we do become central to building enabling environments. In the case of the "Dead Ear Doc," this client never returned, believing that a person so inept at dealing with human beings was likely to miss other vital connections.

PRESENTATION

Therapists who choose to be present and who communicate with integrity convey their approach through the personal context that surrounds them. These people do not require special settings; they are outstanding in whatever situation they find themselves. It is, however, worth considering the visual messages we send to others through our working environments. First impressions matter. Consider how quickly you form an opinion of a store or restaurant that you enter for the first time. When clients enter your working space, what impressions do you think they form? What message are you trying to convey? If you wish to create an enabling environment, what could you do so that the client experiences an enabling environment? Start thinking visually. Look around at the spaces you create around yourself. What do you see? Bulletin boards loaded with tacked-on notes in writing too small to read? Desks stacked with paper and an array of half-finished food and empty coffee cups? Strange looking, and perhaps frightening, equipment all around? The desk positioned as a barrier between the therapist and others? Go into the client-therapist spaces you use and look, as if for the first time. What messages do you receive? If you were to decide to send a visual message to clients, what would it be? Ask clients for their suggestions and comments. If the space looks like a messy teenager works there, consider changing the environment to reflect a professional presentation. Consider replacing the bulletin boards with interesting paintings or posters. Take time to set up a working filing system with hot files for those items you want to keep at hand. Recycle or pack away everything that is never used. Consider organizing and enforcing a system for managing equipment and supplies. Bring life to the area through a few fresh flowers. Create a visually welcoming environment.

For those therapists who go to clients' environments, be sensitive to how you are altering that environment and what message the client reads into changes you are making. The occupational therapist working with a man following his stroke may set up a seemingly useless sanding project on his dining room table without realizing how quickly this foreign device will be packed away, far away from hundreds of warm memories of family celebrations around that table.

Once you have become sensitive to visual messages, consider the auditory messages in the environment. What sort of auditory welcome do clients receive? The loud and abrasive music in the local grocery store sends some of us scurrying to get out of there as fast as possible. What changes can be made in your environment? The warmth of the greetings people receive as they come and go are vital to an enabling environment. Placing the pager on vibrate instead of beep and putting the telephone on call-forward are two examples of changes that can be made. For all therapists, whether we go into client environments or they come into ours, consider the environment where we collect our thoughts. What can we do to make sure it enables our own function?

Having considered the messages clients may read from what they see and hear in the client-therapist space, think about the message your personal presentation makes. How do you convey through your presentation that you are a professional and can be trusted? Not long ago, the author heard someone say, "I took one look at that [professional] and knew he couldn't be trusted." Something went wrong during that initial presentation. We all know people who, without saying a word, present as bristly as porcupines, as open to laughter and play, as overworked and harried, as the expert closed to input, or as the collaborator open to information. Ask a few others to tell you truthfully how you usually present yourself. If you find congruence between how you intend to present, how you are perceived to present, and client-centered practice, then that is validating. However, if you find that people perceive you differently than you intend, or that what you thought was client-centered is not coming across that way, reflect on what you have learned and what you might change without changing who you are.

INTERFACE

Each person's personal environment reflects, among other things, current thinking and feeling, values, and history, although it is not always verbalized. This rich environment is expressed through presence, communication, and presentation. At the point of interface, the personal environments of the therapist and client overlap. This creates a unique environment, that, although part therapist's environment and part client's, becomes shared environment. What we say and what we do influences the personal environments of others, just as they influence ours.

Clients, like therapists, make an impression through their presentation, their presence, and their communication. Ideally, in the occupational therapy process, this interfacing environment contributes to a productive and respectful partnership. The reflective therapist recognizes that the interface between the client's personal environment and the therapist's is not only unique but has the potential to be enabling as well.

Therapist and client expectations and assumptions regarding their time together are important. The therapist who has seen 50 people with the "same" diagnosis may expect to whip through the client-therapist process rapidly. In this way, she is focused on communicating content. The client, on the other hand, may be trying to understand not only what has happened but also why. Typically, the client does not verbalize this thought and feeling process. What is the meaning of this injury, illness, or issue in my life? Did I do something to deserve this? Was it an accident or "divine retribution"? Never mind raised toilet seats or splints (content), what will I do now that the way I am able to be present with others, the way I present, or the way I communicate (context) has changed? How will I do what has meaning to me, and how will I be myself when I do not even know who this different self is? Therapists who record "inability to cope" on clients' health records reveal far more of their own inability to connect than they shed light on client issues. It is too easy to label or make verbal caricatures of people because of one or more unusual behaviors. Labeling is always an indication that the therapist has not seen the meaning behind the presentation. What meaning lies behind the labels "uncooperative" and "unmotivated"? And more significantly, what can the client do to resolve either of these?

In practice, both clients and therapists can present and communicate in ways that either do not connect or that create reaction. When a client needs to be heard and the therapist is feeling too rushed and preoccupied to listen, a "slick boundary" is created. That is, the personal environments slide past each other without engaging and certainly without creating an enabling environment. When the therapist shuts down a client's expression of emotion, a "sticky environment" may be created. That is, the therapist's inability to be present in the moment with emotion can "stick" to the client's self-perception and therefore become part of the client's environment. When a therapist passes a tissue to the weeping client and presses on, an opportunity is missed for the client to experience that it is okay to be him- or herself, that what is felt is important, and that the client is important. Boundaries may be characterized in many different ways. "Phantom boundaries" reflect a lack of judgment as to where personal boundaries end. It is very difficult to get beyond "thick boundaries," which present as boredom and lack of interest. Anyone who has been treated as a body part, such as a hip or knee, will have experienced a thick boundary that prevents therapist understanding of the meaning behind presentation, presence, and communication.

Creating enabling environments is an interactive and deeply reflective process. One exercise that can be useful in increasing awareness of interfacing environments is to observe self and others, both within and outside the therapeutic environment, with the following questions in mind:

1. Who is actively present and who is absent although present? How do you know?
2. Who is complaining and who is truth telling? How do you know? How do responses to complaining and truth telling differ?
3. Who is listening? Is anyone listening? How do you know?
4. Who is asking questions to get to the meaning of comments? How is the questioning done?

This chapter is intended to challenge therapists to care for themselves in such a way that they bring health to every interaction. Healthy and reflective therapists can create and hold space within their personal contexts (hubs) for meaningful human interactions. Through reflection on personal presence, communication, and presentation, therapists can work toward co-creating an enabling environment with each client.

REFERENCES

Arrien, A. (1993). *The four-fold way: Walking the paths of the warrior, teacher, healer and visionary.* San Francisco: Harper.

Canadian Association of Occupational Therapists (CAOT) (1997). *Enabling occupation: An occupational therapy perspective.* Ottawa, Ontario, Canada: CAOT Publications ACE.

Goldstein, J. (1976). *The experience of insight.* Boston: Shambhala Publications, Inc.

Klein, E., & Izzo, J.B. (1999). *Awakening corporate soul: Four paths to unleashing the power of people at work.* Lions Bay, British Columbia, Canada: Fairwinds Press.

Law, M., Cooper, B., Strong, S., Stewart, D., Rigby, P., & Letts, L. (1996). The Person-Environment-Occupation model: A transactive approach to occupational performance. *Canadian Journal of Occupational Therapy, 63,* 9-23.

MacKenzie, G. (1996). *Orbiting the giant hairball: A corporate fool's guide to surviving with grace.* Toronto, Ontario, Canada: Penguin Books, Ltd.

Robinson, V.M. (1991). *Humor and the health professions: The therapeutic use of humor in health care.* (2nd ed.). Thorofare, NJ: SLACK Incorporated.

Ross, R.B. (1994). The ladder of inference. In P.M. Senge, A. Kleiner, C. Roberts, R.B. Ross, & B.J. Smith. *The Fifth Discipline Fieldbook: Strategies and Tools for Building a Learning Organization* (pp. 242-246). New York: Doubleday.

Schaef, A.W. (1998). *Living in process: Basic truths for living the path of the soul.* Toronto, Ontario, Canada: Random House.

Shaeffer, J. (1996). *The stone people: Living together in a different world.* Waterloo, Ontario, Canada: Forsyth Publications.

Strong, S., Rigby, P., Stewart, D., Law, M., Letts, L., & Cooper, B. (1999). Application of the Person-Environment-Occupation Model: A practical tool. *Canadian Journal of Occupational Therapy, 66,* 122-133.

Whyte, D. (1994). *The heart aroused.* New York: Doubleday.

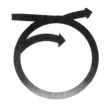

REFLECTING ON CLIENTS IN CONTEXT: A GUIDE TO CLIENT-THERAPIST PARTNERSHIPS USING THE OCCUPATIONAL PERFORMANCE PROCESS MODEL

Introduction to Section II: The Occupational Performance Process Model

Jo Clark, BSc(OT), OT(C)

In Section I of this book, we reflected on the congruence and relationship of leadership values to client-centered values. We continued by examining how we enable or disable through the environments we create. Thus, leadership and enabling environments make up the first portion of the client-centered equation. The remaining variable is a process of occupational therapy that is thorough yet flexible and based on the uniqueness of individuals. The Occupational Performance Process Model (OPPM) (Fearing, Law, & Clark, 1997) provides a guideline for this remaining portion of the equation (see box). Thus,

(OPPM + enabling environments) x leadership = client-centered practice

This section of the book details the seven stages of the OPPM. This model is a dynamic and shared process between clients and therapists. The OPPM suggests a way of being with clients that is initiated by connecting with each individual through his or her story and allowing that story to drive everything else we do in therapy. The model represents a means of reinstating client momentum that may have been lost as a result of occupational performance issues. From identification of issues of importance to the client through to the resolution of these issues, the process is one of equity and partnership.

Although the OPPM is divided into seven different stages representing the various pieces of occupational therapy process, it is best utilized as a guideline for an integrated approach. Because it begins with initial interviews and ends in the measurement of outcomes, it makes the therapist think through every stage of the clinical reasoning process. More than just a list of "how to's," it suggests a nonlinear and flexible process with flow from one stage to another. When using the OPPM, clients and therapists typically begin at Stage 1 and proceed through all of the stages. In some cases, clients and therapists may begin the process in one clinical setting and complete it in another. Or perhaps after beginning in Stage 1, therapists may decide to apply this guideline differently and in a fashion that makes sense given the context and story of the individual.

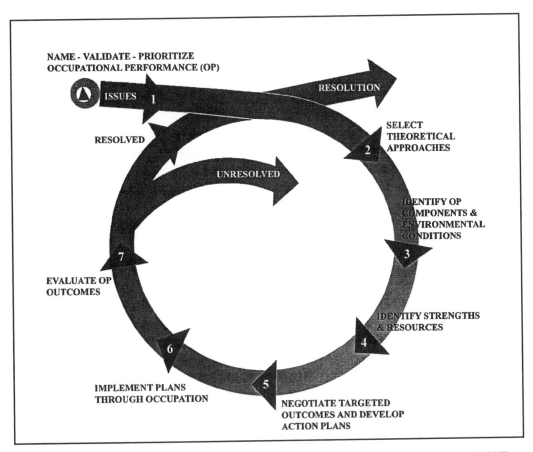

Occupational Performance Process Model. From Fearing, V.G., Law, M., & Clark, J. (1997). An occupational performance process model: Fostering client and therapist alliances. *Canadian Journal of Occupational Therapy, 64*, 11. Reprinted with permission of CAOT Publications.

When used as a guideline, the OPPM does not result in a rigid approach to therapy. Instead, clients and therapists may move back and forth and through the process as judgment indicates. At the end of the seven stages, the process is usually completed with resolution of issues that matter to the client. In the therapy process, if the client is satisfied with performance in desired occupation, and life momentum is once again restored, the process is completed, and the client continues in his or her development. If the client is not satisfied or if other issues are identified, the process can be reinstated by starting at the beginning again or some other stage of the process until satisfaction is achieved.

The OPPM fits with a number of other models. The Canadian Model of Occupational Performance (CMOP) (Canadian Association of Occupational Therapists, 1997) is a conceptual model, which helps us to understand people, the environments in which they live, and the occupations in which they engage. The CMOP defines the elements of occupation (self-care, productivity, leisure), person (components—cognitive, affective, and physical, with spirituality as the core or essence of the individual), and environment (social, physical, cultural, and institutional). The OPPM is a model of practice that guides change and assists individuals to reconnect with desired occupations by understanding and minimizing the components (person) or conditions (environment) that may be obstructing performance.

The Person–Environment–Occupation (PEO) model (Law, Cooper, Strong, Stewart, Rigby, & Letts, 1996) refers to the dynamic connection among these three realms and the resulting performance in occupation. The PEO model guides our thinking related to the assessment and intervention stages of the OPPM. We consider the fit and overlap among meaningful pursuits, personal components, and the contexts in which they take place.

Besides promoting client-centered practice, the OPPM can also be used as a means to organize supporting data and tools. Stage by stage, we can sort, review, and gather evidence that enhances the entire process of occupational therapy (Egan, Dubouloz, von Zweck, & Vallerand, 1998).

Clients pursue occupational therapy service when there is loss of momentum in occupational performance. In the context of this book, some authors refer to occupational performance concerns as issues, others refer to them as problems. Use whatever term clients prefer. The terminology we use throughout the therapy process should be clear and comfortable for clients. Although clients are referred to as individuals, children and their families, or adults and associate clients (the network of people around individuals), the OPPM can also be used with agencies or industry.

The following seven chapters outline the methods and beliefs within each of the stages of the OPPM. The eighth chapter demonstrates the use of the OPPM through a case study, and the ninth chapter explores examples of applications of the OPPM.

REFERENCES

Canadian Association of Occupational Therapists (CAOT). (1997). *Enabling occupation: An occupational therapy perspective.* Ottawa, Ontario, Canada: CAOT Publications ACE.

Egan, M., Dubouloz, C.J., von Zweck, C., & Vallerand, J. (1998). The client-centred evidence-based practice of occupational therapy. *Canadian Journal of Occupational Therapy, 65,* 136-142.

Fearing, V.G., Law, M., & Clark, J. (1997). An occupational performance process model: Fostering client and therapist alliances. *Canadian Journal of Occupational Therapy, 64,* 7-15.

Law, M., Cooper, B., Strong, S., Stewart, D., Rigby, P., & Letts, L. (1996). The Person–Environment–Occupation model: A transactive approach to occupational performance. *Canadian Journal of Occupational Therapy, 63,* 9-23.

chapter three

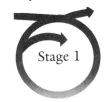

Stage 1

Identifying Occupational Performance Issues

Mary Law, PhD, OT(C)

The first step of the Occupational Performance Process Model (OPPM) (Fearing, Law, & Clark, 1997), identifying occupational performance issues (OPIs), is the focus of this chapter. Through discussion of methods and strategies, and self-reflection about this process, the importance of listening to a client's story, identification of OPIs, and ways to ensure the validity of this process are clarified. This process is similar to a screening process, to identify those issues that are considered by the client to be important and needing occupational therapy intervention. The chapter includes a brief description of screening, methods that can be used to identify OPIs, and a discussion of issues related to the identification process.

LISTENING TO THE CLIENT'S STORY

Think about the last time that you visited a health professional for the first time. You were probably concerned that your issues and questions would be heard and answered. You wanted the person to take the time to hear what you had to say, so that he or she understood your problem. In this situation, you are no different from every client who sees an occupational therapist for the first time. Clients of occupational therapy want to know that you, as their therapist, will listen and hear their concerns.

Consider the following two scenarios, both with the same client. Mrs. MacKay has recently had a cerebral vascular accident, resulting in a stroke affecting the left side of her body. She has come to the rehabilitation center 5 days after the stroke. Her occupational therapist could take different approaches to the initial assessment process (Table 3-1).

Think about these approaches given in Table 3-1. Which is more client-centered? Which process will engage Mrs. MacKay in the therapy process right from the beginning? Which will lead to the identification of the OPIs that are important to Mrs. MacKay?

In the first approach, the therapist begins by listening to the client's story and using the Canadian Occupational Performance Measure (COPM) as the basis to develop an understanding of Mrs. MacKay's current OPIs. By taking the time to hear her story, the therapist learns about her interests, motivations, and the occupations that are causing her

---

Table 3-1
Different Approaches for Initial Assessment Process

Identification of OPIs	Standard Assessment and Intervention Protocol
Therapist talks to Mrs. MacKay to gather information about her life, interests, and occupations of importance to her. Using the COPM, the therapist guides Mrs. MacKay through the identification of OPIs. She identifies self-feeding and holding a book as the two OPIs that are most important to her right now.	Therapist interviews Mrs. MacKay, asking her about her ability to perform basic self-care activities. She says that she is having difficulty moving in and out of bed. The therapist asks about other symptoms resulting from the stroke.
Therapist observes Mrs. MacKay at mealtime and when reading to determine why she is having difficulty performing these tasks. Further analysis of these observations and interventions follows.	Therapist completes an assessment of activities of daily living and a perceptual assessment to gather baseline information prior to intervention.
Other OPIs are identified in the same manner.	Intervention begins, focusing on improving perceptual skills and activities of daily living.

---

difficulty. Through the COPM, these issues are validated with Mrs. MacKay, and the direction for therapy intervention is determined. This approach is very narrative in nature, with the purpose of developing an understanding of Mrs. MacKay in the context in which she lives.

The second approach described in this scenario is more traditional, yet reflects current practice in many locations. While the therapist begins with an interview with Mrs. MacKay, the discussion focuses less on the client's story of her important occupations and more on the resulting symptoms of her stroke. Assessment is not guided by the issues that Mrs. MacKay identified, and intervention centers on improving the performance components (e.g., perception) that underlie performance of occupation.

Therapists generally agree that identification of OPIs is very important in the initial stages of occupational therapy intervention. There is, however, less agreement about the skills required to do this and the most appropriate methods to use. An effective process to identify OPIs requires considerable skill to ensure that rapport is built and that the therapist truly listens to the client's story. Let's look at some of these issues in more detail.

HOW DO I HEAR THE PERSON'S STORY?

Kalmanson and Seligman (1992) state that the "success of all types of interventions will rest on the quality of the relationships between professional providers and family members, even when the relationship itself is not the focus of the intervention" (p. 46). The most

---

Hearing a Person's Story—Questions to Think About

- Do I leave enough time so that clients feel they are able to tell me about the OPIs that are affecting them?
- Am I able to develop an understanding of a person's values after talking to him or her?
- Do I let an interview unfold naturally, rather than structuring each question that I ask of the client? Do I use more open-ended than closed-ended questions?
- Am I observing how the person reacts during the interview and adjusting my interactions based on those observations?
- Do I share my perceptions of what the client has said with him or her to confirm if I am interpreting the information correctly?

---

important act that a therapist can do is to listen and hear the client's story. Persons seeking occupational therapy services are the experts in their lives. They have knowledge about the occupations that are important to them and those with which they are having difficulty. Occupational therapists, on the other hand, bring knowledge about the identification of factors impeding occupational performance and methods that can be used with the client to resolve these issues.

Be careful to avoid professional jargon in establishing a relationship with the person and his or her family. Such jargon works to distance clients from the therapist and discourages them from openly identifying issues for intervention. It is easier to hear a person's story by using open-ended interview questions. There are some situations, though, when more structure is required (e.g., client with recent brain injury). By carefully monitoring the person's reactions during an interview, therapists can be guided by their responses to ensure that the person understands what is being discussed and is feeling comfortable.

WHAT SKILLS DO I NEED AS A THERAPIST?

Client-centered occupational therapy represents a shift from the traditional way of providing occupational therapy service to a method that emphasizes equality, sharing, and partnership. As well, occupational therapists are more frequently providing services to non-health care groups and organizations such as companies, community agencies, and governments. In all of these situations, clients have more power and freedom to make choices that fit with their lives. Occupational therapists facilitate clients to make changes to improve occupational performance. The therapeutic process involves a sharing of control and power.

Occupational therapists need the skills to enable clients to have more control and participate equally in the therapy process. Therapists must be comfortable in engaging in a discussion about the meaning of occupation and the ways in which occupational therapy could assist in resolving OPIs. Clients need support to become confident in developing such a partnership with an occupational therapist. Skills of interaction, negotiation, and facilitation of problem-solving are necessary for a successful client-centered encounter. As service providers in an interview about family-centered service stated:

> *It's individual negotiating. Everyone has [his or her] own style and [his or her] own skills and it's really a matter of trying to come to some level playing ground that everyone can work with.*

> *It's about collaborating and being honest and open about what each of you can offer.* (Law, Brown, Barnes, King, Rosenbaum, & King, 1997)

WHY IS THE CLIENT THE EXPERT?

Clients see occupational therapists for a very short time each day and for short periods in their lives. Recognition of the client's expertise in defining the issue for therapy intervention serves to increase his or her motivation to engage in the therapy process. Acknowledging that the client is the expert regarding personal occupations and providing strategies to identify OPIs promote skills for living. Our goal is to develop the skills that the client has so that occupational therapy is no longer needed.

HOW DO I LEARN ABOUT A PERSON'S OCCUPATIONAL HISTORY?

If you want to learn about a person's occupations, an interview must focus on occupation, not on the components of occupation. For example, if a client comes to you after sustaining a hand injury, and you begin by assessing range of motion and strength, that sends a clear message to the client that those are the outcomes of interest. On the other hand, if you begin by asking the client about everyday occupations in self-care, work, and leisure and difficulties encountered since the hand injury, he or she will understand that the outcome of interest is daily occupation. By doing this, you will gain knowledge from the client about his or her life "in context." There is no one "right" way to identify OPIs but the focus of the identification process centers on performance of occupations rather than performance components or environmental conditions. It is through listening to a client's story that OPIs emerge.

WHY IS IT IMPORTANT TO PRIORITIZE OPIs?

As was stated earlier, clients are the experts on their own lives and are more likely than the therapists to know what is important to them and what will make a difference in their day-to-day lives. Because clients are often not asked to prioritize issues within the health care system, some may be uncomfortable with doing this. It is important to point out that it is only the client and the family who can identify the most important OPIs for them. After that, the expertise of the occupational therapist is used in working together with the client to assess why occupational performance difficulties are occurring and to intervene to increase performance.

IDENTIFICATION OF OPIs—A SCREENING PROCESS?

Screening is used in many health and public health programs to identify risk factors, health problems, or other issues for potential intervention. For example, all of us have seen blood pressure cuff machines in our local drugstore or advertisements for blood pressure screening clinics. The purpose of these measures is to identify persons who have or are at risk for high blood pressure so that problems are identified and an intervention started.

In occupational therapy, screening involves the identification and prioritization of OPIs. When an individual, group, or organization is referred to or seeks out occupational therapy services, the occupational therapist, together with the person or group, seeks to determine if there are issues that require occupational therapy intervention. When using a theoretical approach centered on persons doing occupations within their environment, this determination focuses on whether the person or group is having difficulty in performing occupations of their choice (i.e., occupational performance). The use of such an identification process is both a necessary and efficient way to ensure that occupational therapy services are provided to those who require them. It is unreasonable to assume that everyone seeking out or referred to occupational therapy will require or benefit from the services.

In screening for the need for services, it is important for occupational therapists to do this in a way that is effective and efficient. Guidelines for ensuring the effectiveness of screening programs have been developed (Cadman, Chambers, Feldman, & Sackett, 1984; Sackett, Haynes, Tugwell, & Guyatt, 1996). The following questions can be used by occupational therapists to guide their practice in order to ensure that screening for OPIs is evidence-based and does more good than harm.

Have any studies been completed comparing occupational performance and health outcomes for persons who participated in an occupational performance identification and goal setting process?

Screening identifies those persons, groups, or organizations who are having problems in occupational performance that are affecting their quality of life. Neistadt (1987) and Neistadt and Marques (1984) found that clients who collaborated in the goal-setting process made important gains after occupational therapy intervention in contrast to previous intervention in which the therapists had set the goals by themselves.

Is the OPI of sufficient importance to be identified and receive intervention?

All people, at times in their lives, encounter issues with occupational performance. Some of these issues are serious enough to cause significant disruptions in healthy living while others are not of major consequence. One of the purposes of screening for OPIs is to identify those issues that are serious enough to warrant intervention. It is important to make sure that the screening process is identifying persons or groups who truly have OPIs and screening out those who do not.

Is a screening done consistently and with everyone seeking occupational therapy services?

As a beginning step in the service provision process, screening for OPIs enables clients and therapists to know if further assessment and possible therapy intervention is required. By framing assessment to center on identification of OPIs, therapists will begin to understand the clients' occupations and whether or not they need and are ready for occupational therapy intervention.

If the screening identifies OPIs, is further assessment and intervention available?

It is unfair to screen for issues of importance to the person if adequate intervention services cannot then be provided. The impact of a screening program on resources needs to be determined. As therapists working in health systems with finite resources, we can take the information provided to us by clients about their OPIs and use it to advocate for the development of programs that closely target clients' needs.

If OPIs are identified, can your program offer intervention that is known to be effective?

In developing an evidence-based occupational therapy practice, it is necessary to collect outcome information to support the effectiveness of an occupational therapy service. Such outcome data, along with results from research studies, provide the basis for determining specific programs that will be offered to clients.

WHY IDENTIFY OPIs?

Screening for OPIs, as the beginning step in the OPPM, highlights the importance of taking time to get to know clients and ensuring that occupational therapy services are required in each situation. One part of an evidence-based occupational therapy service is using methods that are effective and efficient in identifying clients who truly require occupational therapy services. Given health care restraints, service should be provided to those for whom intervention can make a difference. In developing new initiatives for groups and organizations in the community, identification of OPIs facilitates program planning and evaluation. Thus, the use of such a screening process serves to improve the effectiveness of future services because occupational therapy is then focused on issues of importance to the client(s) and areas in which change has the potential to lead to important difference in the performance of occupations.

Research on the implementation of client-centered practice has indicated that time is one of the most significant barriers (Law et al., 1997). One of the great advantages of the use of an occupational performance identification process is that it saves time. The majority of clients or their families are able to identify OPIs (McColl, Patterson, Doubt, &

Law, in press). Only those clients who identify OPIs requiring intervention are seen for further assessment and possible intervention, and this saves time. For clients who need intervention, therapy is focused only on issues of importance to the client, thus ensuring efficiency and promoting increased effectiveness.

METHODS TO IDENTIFY OPIs

Several methods have been developed to facilitate a client-centered approach to the identification of OPIs. These methods will only be discussed briefly here, as there are more complete resources available from other sources. For example, Pollock and McColl (1998) outline several methods of assessment of OPIs from a client-centered perspective.

Both qualitative and quantitative assessment methods have been identified as appropriate for use by occupational therapists to screen for OPIs. The methods described here fit with the assumptions articulated by Pollock and McColl (1998) that clients can identify their needs for therapy, that the point of view of the clients regarding OPIs is most important, and that the role of the therapist is to provide intervention that facilitates change.

From a qualitative perspective, the method that is used most often by occupational therapists is an informal interview with the client (Neistadt, 1995). In a survey of occupational therapists working in adult physical rehabilitation facilities, Neistadt (1995) found that the majority of client goals identified through informal interview were vague and did not focus on specific OPIs for intervention. She recommended the use of more structured interview processes for goal identification.

Interviews can be effective, but they are only effective if done in a way that provides structure and guidance to the client in identifying OPIs (Neistadt, 1995; Pollock & McColl, 1998). Some examples of a more structured approach include the use of metaphor, narrative methods, and life histories (Gitlin, Corcoran, & Leinmiller-Eckhardt, 1995; Mattingly, 1991; Spencer, Krefting, & Mattingly, 1993). Through these approaches, therapists are able to engage with the persons, learn about what brings meaning to their lives, and listen to them for the occupations that are important to them and where they are currently having difficulty. The ability to facilitate such storytelling with clients and to analyze the meaning of clients' stories requires skill and sophistication on the part of the therapist. This approach is most appropriate to use with persons who are able to clearly articulate the meaning of occupation in their daily lives. For many persons receiving occupational therapy, this approach may be too unstructured for them, particularly if they have recently acquired a disability. In these situations, use of a guided approach, in which the therapist listens to the client narrative and identifies and probes regarding the occupations that the client is talking about, is more effective.

For a more guided or structured approach to the identification of OPIs, the following measures are suggested.

COPM

The COPM (Law, Baptiste, Carswell, McColl, Polatajko, & Pollock, 1998) has been in use since 1991. It was developed to reflect the philosophy of the Canadian Model of Occupational Performance (Canadian Association of Occupational Therapists [CAOT], 1997). It is an outcome measure designed for use by occupational therapists to identify OPIs and assess client outcomes in self-care, productivity, and leisure (Law et al., 1998). The focus of the COPM is on gathering narrative information from clients about the occupations that they perform in their lives that are currently causing them difficulty. Through the COPM, clients identify those OPIs that they need to, want to, or are expected to do and that they cannot do at the time. Because the COPM is individualized for each client, it is client-centered and incorporates roles and role expectations within the client's own environment. It considers the importance of the occupation to the client. The COPM is designed to help occupational therapists clearly establish occupational performance goals based on clients' perceptions of need and to evaluate clients' perceptions of change in identified areas in occupational performance.

The COPM is administered using a semi-structured interview conducted by the therapist together with the client and/or caregiver. Through the COPM, the therapist is able to hear the client's story about personal occupations. Average time for completion of the COPM is 30 to 40 minutes. The scoring of the COPM (using a 1 to 10 scale) considers the importance, to the client, of the occupational performance areas, as well as the client's current performance and satisfaction with performance. This measure is client-centered, generic (i.e., not diagnosis specific), and crosses developmental stages.

The COPM helps to engage the client from the beginning of the occupational therapy experience and to increase client control of the therapeutic process. As demonstrated in the example of Mrs. MacKay, the COPM aids therapists in soliciting client narration and prioritization of OPIs. It leads to validation of client issues and establishes a baseline against which to measure outcomes (Stage 7).

The 3rd edition of the COPM (Law et al., 1998) is published by the CAOT, Carleton Technology and Training Centre, Suite 3400, 1125 Colonel By Drive, Ottawa, Ontario, Canada K1S 5R1; telephone: 613-523-2268; fax: 613-523-2552; website: www.caot.ca. It is available in the United States through the American Occupational Therapy Association, in Australia through the Australian Association of Occupational Therapists, and in Britain through the College of Occupational Therapy.

OCCUPATIONAL PERFORMANCE HISTORY INTERVIEW (OPHI-II)

The OPHI-II is an assessment of a person's occupational life history in the areas of work, leisure, and daily life activities (Kielhofner & Henry, 1988; Kielhofner et al., 1998). The OPHI-II is administered through an interview by the therapist. Developed using the Model of Human Occupation, the OPHI-II interview focuses on the areas of organization of daily routines, life roles, interests, values and goals, perceptions of ability and responsibility, and environmental influences. The Life History Narrative Form is also included with the OPHI-II and can be used to document qualitative information arising from the interview.

The OPHI-II is designed for use with adolescents, adults, and the elderly and takes an average of 45 to 50 minutes to complete. It can be used in all areas of occupational therapy practice. Scoring is completed by the therapist using a 5-point scale with 1 = maladaptation and 5 = adaptation. The OPHI-II has been found to aid therapists in establishing rapport, identifying problems, and setting therapy goals.

The OPHI-II is available through the American Occupational Therapy Association, 4720 Montgomery Lane, Bethesda, MD 20814-3425; telephone: 301-652-2682; fax: 301-652-7711; website: www.aota.org.

OCCUPATIONAL SELF ASSESSMENT (OSA)

The OSA is a new assessment based on the work of the *Self Assessment of Occupational Functioning*, developed by Baron and Curtin (1990). The OSA is designed to be an evaluation tool that assesses personal perception of occupational competence and the environmental influences on occupational adaptation. Persons completing the OSA first rate how well they are functioning on each item and then rate the importance of the area of functioning or environmental influence for each item. Items that are rated low in functioning and are perceived to be important to the person are considered for occupational therapy intervention.

The OSA is a self-report assessment completed by the person seeking occupational therapy services. The occupational competence section assesses occupational performance, habituation, and volition, while the environmental section assesses physical and social environments. This assessment can be used with clients of all ages and diagnoses. The results of the OSA are designed to be used by the therapist and client to decide a course of occupational therapy intervention. Because the OSA includes a set list of items, its ability to provide individualized information about a client in context may be limited. Time to complete the OSA has not been reported.

Contact the Model of Human Occupation Clearinghouse, Department of Occupational Therapy (MC 811), College of Associated Health Professions, 1919 West Taylor Street, Chicago, IL 60612-7250; fax: 312-413-0256 for more information on *The Occupational Self Assessment User's Manual* (Baron, Kielhofner, Goldhammer, & Wolenski, 1999).

WHEN IS THE BEST TIME TO IDENTIFY OPIs?

Identification of OPIs works best if done as an initial assessment. Learning about the client's issues from his or her perspective right from the beginning signals to the client that this will be a working partnership. It ensures that the therapist takes the time to connect with clients and learn about their needs. As well, knowing the client's priorities helps the therapists to focus further assessment and intervention on the components contributing to OPIs rather than a general assessment approach based on diagnosis.

HOW DO I IDENTIFY OPIs
FOR GROUPS AND ORGANIZATIONS?

The identification of issues with groups or organizations is more difficult than working with a single client. In identifying issues for occupational therapy intervention with the group, it is important to know if the perspective you receive is that of the group or only a few individuals. Stanton, Kramer, and Thompson-Franson (1997) recommend that a needs assessment be performed to identify OPIs affecting the group and if intervention is required. A needs assessment can be completed using interviews, focus groups, or through a survey. Some of the methods discussed earlier, such as the COPM and the OSA, can also be used to identify common OPIs within a group. This is done by interviewing persons individually and summarizing the results. If the organization is the client, this process will be completed with a person or persons acting as the representative of the organization.

WHAT IF I DO NOT HAVE TIME
TO SCREEN FOR OPIs?

As stated earlier, time is seen as one of the most significant constraints in the implementation of a client-centered practice. There is a perception that the time that is required to engage the client in identification of OPIs and to hear the client's story is more than most therapists have available. It is true that there are some situations (e.g., in an acute-care hospital) where the identification of OPIs needs to be done in a very focused and timely fashion. In most situations, however, the identification of individualized and prioritized OPIs leads to a streamlined occupational therapy assessment and intervention process. Further assessment of performance components and environmental conditions is focused only on issues that have been identified. Intervention then centers on problem-solving related to the most important OPIs. A client's motivation to engage in the intervention process and to change is increased because the intervention has meaning.

WHAT IF THE PERSON
CANNOT OR DOES NOT IDENTIFY ANY OPIs?

There will be occasions when clients are not able to or do not identify any OPIs. When this occurs, it is important to discern whether lack of identification of issues is due to lack of understanding of the process or because there are no issues for which occupational therapy intervention is required. When a client is having difficulty understanding the identification process, a therapist can talk to the family or others within his or her environment to identify these issues. If this is done, it is important to remember that you are obtaining their perceptions rather than the perceptions of the client. If it is clear that the client has understood the process and states that there are no issues that are important, the assessment process will then end. If no issues are identified, further assessment or occupational therapy intervention is not required. It may be that the client has no OPIs or perhaps is not ready to seek intervention at this time.

There will be situations in which the client identifies no OPIs yet there are issues apparent to the therapist. If a client is competent, the fact that no OPIs are identified may reflect personal values and priorities at the moment. It is important in these situations to consider whether these differences in opinion reflect differences in values or issues of the client's competency. The therapist can, and should, point out that the therapist or others believe that the client does have OPIs that require intervention. If the client does not agree with this, is competent to make that decision, and does not desire therapy intervention, the therapist respects this decision. The opportunity for therapy at a later date, if desired, can be communicated to the client.

HOW DO I IDENTIFY OPIs IN PRACTICE SITUATIONS THAT ARE SHORT-LIVED?

There are practice situations in which therapists see clients for very short periods of time (e.g., acute care facilities). In these situations, the methods that have been described to identify OPIs can be used but must be done in a more focused manner. For example, an interview could center on the OPIs that are affecting the person immediately. One way of gathering this information is to ask the person or caregivers/supports what daily living task is causing the most difficulty at the moment. Using this strategy, intervention can focus on issues that will make the most immediate difference to the person in the context of a life in process. Use of the COPM in this situation will identify those immediate issues, and this information can be passed along to other therapists who may be involved with the client as rehabilitation continues, thus making transitions seamless.

WHAT IF A PERSON DOES NOT IDENTIFY SOMETHING THAT I BELIEVE IS IMPORTANT OR I DON'T AGREE WITH WHAT HE OR SHE HAS IDENTIFIED?

As an occupational therapist, there will be situations in which you observe OPIs that are not identified by the client. It is important to discover if these differences are based on different perceptions of the person's occupations, differences in values, or if the person is not able to identify these issues because of lack of insight or other cognitive impairments. It is always important not to make assumptions about a person's level of insight. If the issue that the therapist has identified is an issue of safety or risk, it is the responsibility of the therapist as a professional to discuss that issue with the client and/or caregivers and to take the necessary steps to ensure that the issue is addressed. If the issue does not relate to risk or safety, the best course is to discuss it with the client, and then accept the priorities of the client as the other issues may be raised later. As stated in Law et al. (1997), "You might as well figure out how your goal can be incorporated into theirs, because they just won't work on it, that's not their priority."

DOES THIS IDENTIFICATION PROCESS WORK WITH PEOPLE FROM ALL CULTURES?

It is necessary to remember that the OPPM and the concepts underlying a client-centered practice were developed largely in North America. Because of this, there are implicit assumptions built into these models that are reflective of culture (Iwama, 1999). For example, in North American culture, disability is often viewed as something to be pitied, and independence for people with and without disabilities is highly valued. Views of disability and independence may be quite different in other cultures around the world or in persons of different cultures living in another country. Identification of OPIs should be able to accommodate such differences in values. For example, it may be considered inappropriate for the person who is ill or has a disability to set specific occupational goals for him- or herself. In this situation, the therapist would want to include family members in this discussion so that the OPIs are identified by the whole family and fit with their lifestyle.

The choice of which assessment tool to use in the identification of OPIs is also affected by culture. Although North American, Australian, and European cultures are used to and usually quite comfortable with a numerical rating scale, for many cultures the idea of using numbers to rate items is foreign. In these situations, therapists can use alternative rating scales, for example, a series of frowning to smiling faces, or simply identify the OPIs without a numerical rating. An alternative to using a numerically based assessment tool is to use qualitative methods, such as narrative storytelling, to gain information about the OPIs that are important to the client.

SUMMARY

I asked you at the beginning of this chapter to think about the last time that you visited a health professional for the first time. Now that you have read this chapter, reflect on that experience again. Did the health professional listen to your story, hear your concerns, and consider you to be the expert regarding your health? Did he or she help you to prioritize your concerns? These are the most important issues that are addressed in this chapter. Together, we have explored the importance of listening to the client's story, using valid methods to identify OPIs, and other challenges in the first stage of occupational therapy intervention. As you can see, the process of identification of OPIs lays the groundwork for everything that follows in the occupational therapy service process. The ability to engage with a client to identify issues for potential intervention ensures that further services will be focused and efficient. Such identification also provides the basis for the evaluation of outcomes after occupational therapy services have been received. Taking the necessary time for this stage of the occupational therapy process is critical to everything that follows.

REFERENCES

Baron, K., & Curtin, C. (1990). *Self-assessment of occupational functioning.* Chicago: Model of Human Occupation Clearing House.

Baron, K., Kielhofner, G., Goldhammer, T., & Wolenski, J. (1999). *The Occupational Self Assessment user's manual.* Chicago: University of Chicago.

Cadman, D., Chambers, L., Feldman, W., & Sackett, D. (1984). Assessing the effectiveness of community screening program. *Journal of the American Medical Association, 251,* 1580-1585.

Canadian Association of Occupational Therapists (CAOT) (1997). *Enabling occupation: An occupational therapy perspective.* Ottawa, Ontario, Canada: CAOT Publications ACE.

Fearing, V.G., Law, M., & Clark, J. (1997). An occupational performance process model: Fostering client and therapist alliances. *Canadian Journal of Occupational Therapy, 64,* 7-15.

Gitlin, L., Corcoran, M., & Leinmiller-Eckhardt, S. (1995). Understanding the family perspective: An ethnographic framework for providing occupational therapy in the home. *American Journal of Occupational Therapy, 49,* 802-809.

Iwama, M. (1999). Cross-cultural perspectives on client-centred occupational therapy practice: A view from Japan. *Occupational Therapy Now, Nov/Dec,* 4-6.

Kalmanson, B., & Seligman, S. (1992). Family-provider relationships: The basis of all interventions. *Infants and Young Children, 4,* 46-52.

Kielhofner, G., & Henry, A. (1988). Development and investigation of the Occupational Performance History Interview. *American Journal of Occupational Therapy, 42,* 489-498.

Kielhofner, G., Mallinson, T., Crawford, D., Nowak, M., Rigby, M., Henry, A., & Walens, D. (1998). *Occupational Performance History Interview (OPHI-II).* Bethesda, MD: American Occupational Therapy Association.

Law, M., Baptiste, S., Carswell, A., McColl, M.A., Polatajko, H., & Pollock, N. (1998). *The Canadian Occupational Performance Measure (COPM)* (3rd ed.). Ottawa, Ontario, Canada: CAOT Publications.

Law, M., Brown, S., Barnes, S., King, G., Rosenbaum, P., & King, S. (1997). *Implementing family-centred services in Ontario children's rehabilitation services.* Hamilton, Ontario, Canada: Neurodevelopmental Clinical Research Unit.

Mattingly, C. (1991). The narrative nature of clinical reasoning. *American Journal of Occupational Therapy, 45,* 998-1005.

McColl, M.A., Patterson, M., Doubt, L., & Law, M. (In press.) Validation of the COPM for community practice. *Canadian Journal of Occupational Therapy.*

Neistadt, M.E. (1987). An occupational therapy program for adults with developmental disabilities. *American Journal of Occupational Therapy, 41,* 433-438.

Neistadt, M.E. (1995). Methods of assessing clients' priorities: A survey of adult physical dysfunction settings. *American Journal of Occupational Therapy, 49,* 428-436.

Neistadt, M.E., & Marques, K. (1984). An independent living skills training program. *American Journal of Occupational Therapy, 38,* 671-676.

Pollock, N., & McColl, M.A. (1998). Assessment in client-centred occupational therapy. In M. Law (Ed.), *Client-Centered Occupational Therapy.* Thorofare, NJ: SLACK Incorporated.

Sackett, D., Haynes, B., Tugwell, P., & Guyatt, G. (1996). *Clinical epidemiology.* Oxford, England: Oxford Press.

Spencer, J., Krefting, L., & Mattingly, C. (1993). Incorporation of ethnographic methods in occupational therapy assessment. *American Journal of Occupational Therapy, 47,* 303-309.

Stanton, S., Kramer, C., & Thompson-Franson, T. (1997). Linking concepts to a process for organizing occupational therapy services. In Canadian Association of Occupational Therapists, *Enabling Occupation: An Occupational Therapy Perspective.* Ottawa, Ontario, Canada: CAOT Publications ACE.

chapter four

Stage 2

SELECTING A THEORETICAL APPROACH

MARY ANN McCOLL, PhD, OT(C)

INTRODUCTION

The selection of a theoretical approach is the second step of the Occupational Performance Process Model (OPPM) (Fearing, Law, & Clark, 1997). In the first step, occupational performance problems were identified, using an assessment like the Canadian Occupational Performance Measure (COPM) (Law, Baptiste, Carswell, McColl, Polatajko, & Pollock, 1998). The COPM identifies problems as occupations that the client wants to do, needs to do, or is expected to do, but can't do, doesn't do, or isn't satisfied with the way they are done. In the next step, the occupational therapist begins to figure out how to think about those problems. This process of thinking about occupational performance problems is synonymous with selecting a theoretical approach. It begins with generating hypotheses about the origins of problems and ends with identifying appropriate assessment and intervention approaches.

Occupational therapy theory provides us with ways of thinking about occupation and about the kinds of things that can interfere with occupation. Theory is probably most easily understood as a **tool for thinking**. Following the metaphor, one's store of theory knowledge can then be thought of as a toolbox, from which one selects the most appropriate tool for the job. Just like in carpentry, it is possible to use a number of different tools to do the same job; however, the correct tool makes the job easier. And different workers will have preferences for particular tools with which they are most comfortable and familiar.

In the same way, the broad array of occupational therapy theory is the toolbox from which occupational therapists select ideas, concepts, and principles that help them to understand and influence the occupational performance problems they see in their clients. Some theories are more appropriate for specific occupational performance problems than others. And most occupational therapists have their favorite theoretical approaches. The choice of a favorite theoretical approach may be influenced by a number of factors, such as the area in which one practices, the theoretical approaches used by colleagues, the theories that were prevalent when one was educated, and the accessibility of particular theoretical literature, workshops, or continuing education opportunities.

THE OCCUPATIONAL THERAPY TOOLBOX: TYPES OF OCCUPATIONAL THERAPY THEORY

Our occupational therapy toolbox is separated into two main sections: tools to help us understand occupation and tools to help us change or remediate occupation. The former offers us ways to think, and the latter offers us ways to act. We typically call these two main categories of theory **conceptual models** and **models of practice**. Conceptual models help us to think about occupation, and models of practice help us act therapeutically to change occupation.

The occupational therapy toolbox, or knowledge base, is further divided into theory that is explicitly about occupation and theory that is generally about human beings. We will refer to these as Level I and Level II theory. Level I theory is specifically about occupational performance, and it is most often developed by occupational therapists. It attempts to explain occupation as a function of a variety of other factors, about which we will say more in the next section. Level II theory is all of the other theory, usually from other disciplines, that we learn and use to help us understand human beings. For example, our anatomy, physiology, biology, pathology, kinesiology, and other basic biomedical sciences help us to understand the physical aspect of the human being.

The occupational therapy toolbox therefore begins to look like the matrix in Figure 4-1.

1. Theory located in Section 1 of the toolbox includes conceptual models that help us to understand occupation and the factors that interfere with occupation to produce occupational performance problems. For example, theories about how occupation is acquired and how developmental factors can affect the acquisition of occupation would be found in this section—Level I conceptual models.

2. Theory found in Section 2 includes conceptual models from other disciplines that help us to understand human beings in general. These do not deal specifically with human occupation, but rather with the components of people and environments (which admittedly influence occupation). For example, Level II conceptual models about how muscles receive messages from the central nervous system to produce human movement would be found in Section 2 of the occupational therapy toolbox.

3. Theory found in Section 3 includes occupational therapy models of practice. This is theory that helps us to know how to act to help clients to improve their occupational performance. As an example, theory about how the environment may be modified to enhance occupation would be found in Section 3, on Level I models of practice.

4. Finally, theory found in Section 4 of the matrix includes models of practice relating to specific components of human beings. For example, theory about how occupational therapists might intervene with physical modalities to promote activity tolerance and endurance would be considered a Level II model of practice.

	LEVEL I	LEVEL II
CONCEPTUAL MODELS	1. LEVEL I CONCEPTUAL: Ways of thinking about occupation	2. LEVEL II CONCEPTUAL: Ways of understanding human beings
MODELS OF PRACTICE	3. LEVEL I APPLIED: Ways of acting therapeutically to change occupation	4. LEVEL II APPLIED Ways of acting to change specific components of humans

Figure 4-1. The occupational therapy toolbox.

THE OCCUPATIONAL THERAPY FILING CABINET: THE CONTENT OF OCCUPATIONAL THERAPY THEORY

Up to this point, we have talked about the purposes of theory—to understand humans and their occupation and to be able to help to change human functioning and occupational performance. Now let us turn our attention to the specific content of theory used by occupational therapists.

In order to organize the theory of occupational therapy according to content, we have observed that the theoretical literature on occupation most commonly identifies occupation as a function of the person on one hand and the environment on the other (Canadian Association of Occupational Therapists [CAOT], 1997; Law, Cooper, Strong, Stewart, Rigby, & Letts, 1996; McColl, 1998; McColl, Law, & Stewart, 1992). The person is typically described in terms of interrelated components, each of which has a body of theory associated with it. The most common components used to describe the person include: physical, psychological-emotional, cognitive-neurological, sociocultural, and developmental (CAOT, 1981; McColl et al., 1992; Reed, 1984).

- The **physical** component of the person refers to motor, sensory, proprioceptive, and kinesthetic capacities.
- The **psychological-emotional** component refers to both intrinsic and learned responses of individuals to internal and external stimuli.
- The **cognitive-neurological** component refers to the central processing of internal and external stimuli.
- The **sociocultural** component includes learned beliefs, attitudes, roles, and behaviors that are a result of socialization or upbringing. Meaning and spirituality may be considered parts of the sociocultural component.
- The **developmental** component of the person is made up of the skills, tasks, challenges, and attitudes associated with growth and development.

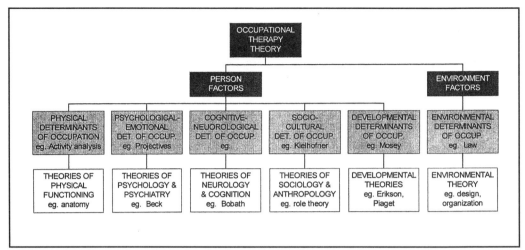

Figure 4-2. Six areas and two levels of occupational therapy theory.

The occupational therapy literature also defines occupation as a function of the **environment**, defined broadly to include both the physical and the social environments.

Throughout our careers, first as students then as occupational therapists, we continually acquire knowledge about all six areas concerning humans and their occupations. However, we do not always have a way of storing this knowledge so that it is readily accessible and usable. We suggest another metaphor to illustrate how occupational therapists might store occupational therapy theory: the filing cabinet. Think about a filing cabinet with six drawers, corresponding to the six theory areas just described (physical, psychological-emotional, cognitive-neurological, sociocultural, developmental, and environmental). In each drawer are four folders, one corresponding to each of the four quadrants of the toolbox or the four types of tools used by occupational therapists (see Figure 4-1): Level I conceptual, Level I applied, Level II conceptual, and Level II applied.

We contend that all of the ideas and theories used by occupational therapists can be readily classified in this filing system. Figure 4-2 gives a summary of how the system might work. We can classify all of our basic occupational therapy education in the 12 boxes of Figure 4-2. Further, we can classify information that we have gained through our experiences as occupational therapists: continuing education, workshops, journals, books, and experience, particularly interactions with other professionals, clients, and their families.

We have talked up to this point about classifying theory, so that it is more readily available to us. Now let us talk about how we can actually use theory. Perhaps the best way to illustrate the utility of this filing system is with an example. The following example shows how we can use theory from all six categories of occupational therapy theory to help us to understand:
- The occupational performance problem faced by the client
- The corresponding problems in underlying components of the person and the environment
- How we might intervene to improve the functioning of a particular component
- How we might intervene to improve occupational performance directly

CASE EXAMPLE

Lisa is a 27-year-old woman who has experienced a depressive reaction following the birth of her second child. She returned home after the birth of her new baby, and within 2 weeks, she was readmitted to mental health services. At that time, she was uncommunicative, emotional, and withdrawn. Her mother has come to stay and is looking after the new baby and the 2-year-old while Lisa is in the hospital. Lisa has 6 months of maternity leave before returning to her job as a legal secretary. Her discharge is planned for the end of the week, and everyone is wondering how Lisa will manage at home. In particular, there is concern about how Lisa will fulfill the occupational requirements of caring for her children. An occupational therapy assessment is requested.

From the **physical** theory perspective, Lisa's potential to fulfill her responsibilities at home would be seen primarily as a function of her stamina and ability to cope with the physical demands of parenting two small children. The occupational therapy assessment would focus on Lisa's ability to sustain an appropriate level of activity for the tasks that she must accomplish. Occupational therapy intervention might focus on physical activity to increase Lisa's activity tolerance, recognizing that physical activity has psychological as well as physical benefits.

From the **psychological-emotional** theory perspective, we would seek to understand Lisa's thoughts and feelings associated with returning home and resuming the care of her children. Assessment would focus on how these feelings were interfering with Lisa's occupation and possibly on the origins of these feelings and ideas. Occupational therapy intervention would address the feelings, perhaps attempting to raise them to a higher level of consciousness and to problem-solve methods for preventing them from interfering.

According to **cognitive-neurological** theory, Lisa's problems would be understood as potentially related to problems in processing incoming information, cognitively, perceptually, or neurologically. It would be important to observe Lisa's capacity to process incoming information, to ensure that there was no neurological problem underlying Lisa's reaction to her situation. It is unlikely that there would be intervention, unless a specific problem was identified.

The **sociocultural** theory area offers another way to understand and address Lisa's occupational performance issues. Lisa's problems may be understood as a function of conflict with her role as a mother, wife, worker, daughter, and so on. Assessment would focus on Lisa's beliefs about the roles she plays, her expectations of herself in those roles, and her perceptions about the expectations of other key players. Occupational therapy intervention would seek to address her issues by attempting to reconcile role expectations and understand role behaviors.

From the **developmental** perspective, Lisa's potential problems would be understood as inadequate development for the challenges at hand. The developmental assessment would focus on the challenges perceived in the environment and the developmental skills required to meet them. Developmental therapy would begin at the level at which

Lisa is currently functioning and would attempt to present Lisa with challenges that would enhance her development through succeeding stages until she had acquired the necessary aptitudes to meet the demands at home.

Finally, from the **environmental** perspective, Lisa's problems would be understood in terms of the ability of her environment to support her in her occupation. Assessment would focus on the physical environment (i.e., the home itself) and the social environment (i.e., Lisa's husband, mother, friends, neighbors, community services). Assessment would attempt to determine what supports and barriers the environment presented, and intervention would attempt to enhance supports and remove barriers.

The example illustrates a number of points:

1. It shows that there are many different ways to approach any occupational performance problem. You may have thought of others that we have not presented.

2. It shows that ways of approaching occupational performance problems can be classified into the six theory areas that we have suggested.

3. The example shows that some ways of understanding a particular problem are more appropriate than others. For example, in our opinion, the psychological-emotional, sociocultural, and environmental approaches offer the most promise of achieving a meaningful understanding of Lisa's situation and of intervening in an effective manner. For therapists with a distinct preference and expertise in a particular theory area, the example shows how it is possible for that theory area to be applicable across a broad spectrum of clients and occupational performance problems. However, such therapists may also recognize that there are instances where that theory is not optimally effective. They then have the responsibility either to use a different theoretical approach or refer to another therapist who will.

4. The example shows how assessment and intervention dovetail within a particular theory area.

5. Finally, the example raises the issue of the boundaries of each of the theory areas. In practice, it is uncommon for a therapist to practice using ideas from only one theory area. More often, we combine ideas and principles from a variety of theory areas. We often refer to this as an eclectic approach to practice. There is nothing wrong with an eclectic approach to practice, as long as it is not a euphemism for an atheoretical approach, based on common sense or intuition. To ensure that this is not the case, it is important to be able to identify the origins of particular ideas that contribute to one's eclectic approach and to ensure that the principles used or the assumptions underlying them are not fundamentally conflicting.

THE PROCESS OF USING
OCCUPATIONAL THERAPY THEORY

The last section of this chapter seeks to incorporate all that we have talked about up to this point into the process of occupational therapy. In other words, we will talk about using the toolbox and the filing cabinet in everyday practice.

The preceding chapter has discussed ways to assess and identify occupational performance problems (see Chapter 3). Once problems are identified, the therapist then begins the process of generating hypotheses about the possible origin of problems. In order to intervene effectively, we must know not only what the problems are, but we must have hypotheses about what factors caused the problems, what factors reinforce and sustain the problems, and what factors can be altered to potentially remediate the problems.

This process of generating hypotheses about factors affecting occupational performance problems leads us directly to the first quadrant of the toolbox—Level I conceptual models. Level I conceptual models provide us with an understanding of the factors affecting occupational performance. In other words, this quadrant contains theory about the relationships between occupational performance problems and components of humans and environments.

Alternatively, we may say that the process of generating hypotheses for the origins of occupational performance problems leads us to the top drawer of the filing cabinet. In much the same way as we did in our example with Lisa, occupational therapists every day rifle through the six folders in the top drawer of their mental filing cabinet to generate hypotheses about why people are experiencing the problems they see. Is there a physical impediment to occupation? Do thoughts or feelings (psychological-emotional), beliefs or values (sociocultural), skills or maturity (developmental) interfere with occupation? Is there a central processing problem that prevents the smooth transition between receiving sensory input and producing occupational output (cognitive-neurological)? Do the physical and social environments adequately support the occupation of the individual? Theory about each of these six areas will help us to develop several working hypotheses about the factors contributing to difficulties with occupational performance.

To follow on with Lisa's example, our hypotheses are that there may be thoughts and feelings (psychological-emotional theory), beliefs about roles (sociocultural theory), or environmental impediments (environmental theory) contributing to Lisa's occupational performance problems. Therefore, our hypotheses might look like this:

- Lisa has depressive ideas, fears of failure, negative thoughts about the self, and low self-esteem, all of which are potentially important determinants of occupational performance.
- Lisa's occupational performance is impaired because she has internalized beliefs about the role of a mother and wife that she does not believe she can fulfill.
- Lisa is receiving messages from her environment that she is expected to function up to a very high standard as a mother, but is not receiving the required support to do so.

Classical occupational therapy theory about analyzing activities for their psychological requirements might help us to explain the problems in Lisa's occupational performance. Theory from Kielhofner's (1985) model of the relationships of roles, values, and habits to occupational performance might also be useful here. Law's (1991) conceptualization of the environment and its impact on occupation might help us to understand the role of the environment in Lisa's difficulties.

To develop a fuller and more detailed understanding of each of these hypotheses, occupational therapists rely on theory about humans and their environments, usually originating in other disciplines. For example, to elaborate on the first hypothesis pertaining to Lisa, we might consult our psychology and psychiatry background to fill in what we know about postpartum depression and the psychological demands of caring for children. For the second hypothesis, we might consult our Level II conceptual models from sociology for information about roles and role conflict. And for the third hypothesis, we might consult our background theory from anthropology to better understand the environmental supports that can assist in sustaining women at home with children.

In order to confirm one or more of these hypotheses, and to gather more evidence about the nature of occupational performance problems, occupational therapists next proceed to find out more about the functioning of specific performance components underlying the most promising hypotheses. To understand the nature and extent of underlying problems, they rely on Level II models of practice to suggest appropriate assessments of human performance components and of the environment.

In our example, we might use a depression inventory, a self-esteem measure, an unstructured interview about ideas and emotions associated with discharge and return home, a role inventory, a measure of role conflict, a home assessment, a support inventory, and unstructured interviews with other key personnel, such as husband and mother.

Armed with all of this information and a thorough understanding of the nature, extent, and probable origins of the occupational performance problems, the therapist is finally ready to share the results of his or her assessment with the client and to work together to set goals and select therapeutic approaches to remediate occupational performance problems. For this task, he or she relies on Level I models of practice to offer guidance for therapeutic approaches to occupational performance problems in each of the six areas.

SUMMARY AND CONCLUSION

The chapter uses two metaphors—the toolbox and the filing cabinet—to describe how occupational therapists use theory. Theory is needed in occupational therapy to help us to think about humans and their occupations (conceptual models) and to intervene to make changes in the person, his or her occupation, and the environment (models of practice). Further, six theory areas are found in the occupational therapy literature, each elaborating how a different aspect of humans or environments relates to occupation. Through an example, we have explored the potential of occupational therapy theory to explain occupational dysfunction and to direct us as to how to proceed in assessment and treatment. The next chapter proceeds to discuss assessment to identify which of the six areas of theory is most applicable for a particular client.

ACKNOWLEDGMENTS

The author acknowledges Mary Law, Debra Stewart, and Lorna Doubt for contributions to earlier works involving some of the ideas in this chapter.

REFERENCES

Canadian Association of Occupational Therapists (CAOT) (1981). *Guidelines for the client-centred practice of occupational therapy*. Toronto, Ontario, Canada: CAOT Publications.

Canadian Association of Occupational Therapists (CAOT) (1997). *Enabling occupation: An occupational therapy perspective*. Ottawa, Ontario, Canada: CAOT Publications ACE.

Fearing, V.G., Law, M., & Clark, J. (1997). An occupational performance process model: Fostering client and therapist alliances. *Canadian Journal of Occupational Therapy, 64*, 7-15.

Kielhofner, G. (1985). *A model of human occupation: Theory and applications*. Baltimore: Williams & Wilkins.

Law, M. (1991). The environment: A focus for occupational therapy. *Canadian Journal of Occupational Therapy, 58*(4), 171-179.

Law, M., Baptiste, S., Carswell, A., McColl, M.A., Polatajko, H., & Pollock, N. (1998). *The Canadian Occupational Performance Measure (COPM)* (3rd ed.). Ottawa, Ontario, Canada: CAOT Publications.

Law, M., Cooper, B., Strong, S., Stewart, D., Rigby, P., & Letts, L. (1996). The Person-Environment-Occupation model: A transactive approach to occupational performance. *Canadian Journal of Occupational Therapy, 63*, 9-23.

McColl, M.A. (1998). What do we need to know to practice occupational therapy in the community? *American Journal of Occupational Therapy, 52*(1), 11-18.

McColl, M.A., Law, M., & Stewart, D. (1992). *Theoretical basis of occupational therapy*. Thorofare, NJ: SLACK Incorporated.

Reed, K.L. (1984). *Models of practice in occupational therapy*. Baltimore: Williams & Wilkins.

chapter five

Stage 3

IDENTIFYING PERFORMANCE COMPONENTS AND ENVIRONMENTAL CONDITIONS CONTRIBUTING TO OCCUPATIONAL PERFORMANCE ISSUES

CATHERINE BACKMAN, MS, OT(C), NONIE MEDCALF, BSc(OT), OT(C)

Imagine going into a department store and having the salesperson sell you a sofa when what you really wanted was new carpet for your living room. This is akin to an occupational therapist assessing a client's functional status before listening to the client's story and hearing what occupational performance issues (OPIs) are most important at that point in time. Like the dissatisfied shopper who brushes off the salesperson, clients may lose their desire to participate in the occupational therapy process if they feel their concerns are not heard or it appears that time will be wasted on unimportant problems. That's why two stages in the Occupational Performance Process Model (OPPM) precede the stage described in this chapter; if you skipped them, you might want to back up!

Once initial OPIs have been identified with the client and appropriate theoretical approaches have been determined (Chapters 3 and 4), the next step is to investigate possible underlying causes of dysfunction or difficulties giving rise to the OPIs. Just like an attentive sales consultant finds out about product requirements, price range, and colors, a client-centered occupational therapist works with the client to identify preferences. Specifically, the occupational therapist considers characteristics within individuals, their environments, and the interaction between the two that contribute to the initial OPIs. In this chapter, we will discuss the implementation of Stage 3 in the OPPM (Fearing, Law, & Clark, 1997), that of identifying performance components (the client's skills and abilities) and the environmental conditions relevant to the OPIs identified by the client.

DEFINITIONS FOR THIS CHAPTER

Terms used in this chapter are consistent with those defined in the Canadian Model of Occupational Performance (Townsend et al., 1997). Table 5-1 contains definitions of

---

Table 5-1
Definitions of Key Terms

Occupational performance:	The ability to choose, organize, and satisfactorily perform meaningful occupations.
Performance components:	Characteristics or skills possessed by a person that enable occupational performance.
1. Affective (feeling):	Social and emotional function.
2. Cognitive (thinking):	Mental and intellectual functions such as perception, concentration, comprehension, judgment, and reasoning.
3. Physical (doing):	Sensation and motor function.
Environmental conditions:	Elements of the environment that may enhance or hinder a person's ability to perform.
1. Cultural:	Ceremonial and routine practices based on ethos and value systems of a particular group.
2. Institutional:	Societal institutions and practices, including policies and legislation.
3. Physical:	Natural and built surroundings (e.g., weather, buildings, roads).
4. Social:	Patterns of relationships of people living in an organized community, social groups based on common interests, values, attitudes, and beliefs.

Adapted from Townsend et al. (1997). *Enabling occupation: An occupational therapy perspective.* Ottawa, Ontario, Canada: CAOT Publications.

---

key terms. OPIs arise when there is dysfunction or dissatisfaction with occupational performance. Performance components and environmental conditions (consistent with the hypotheses generated in Stage 2) then become the focus of assessment. For the purposes of this chapter, assessment is "the process of collecting, analyzing, and interpreting information, obtained through observation, interview, record review, and testing" (Canadian Association of Occupational Therapists, 1991, p. 137). As limitations in performance components and environmental conditions are identified, the client and therapist can reflect on these findings and validate or reject them as the underlying causes of the client's OPIs.

GETTING STARTED

The process outlined in Chapter 3 has already initiated a client-centered relationship: an interview has taken place, rapport has been established, and the client's priorities have been elicited. We know that the client has identified one or more OPIs; otherwise, we would not have progressed to subsequent stages in the OPPM "loop." A theoretical approach was selected in Chapter 4, which guides how we think about occupation in the context of a particular client's life, and we have some idea about which theories could be employed to guide the collection of more data. In this chapter, we want to build upon the relationship already initiated and apply the theoretical approaches selected in Stage 2 as we gather additional data. These data will validate the OPIs, provide baseline information against which change may be assessed, and direct subsequent stages in the occupational performance process.

Pollock and McColl (1998) refer to assessment as a two-tiered process of problem identification and problem analysis. The identification of OPIs has already resulted in some data related to identification of problems that indicate the need for occupational therapy (tier one); analysis of potential causes of dysfunction must then be sorted out (tier two). Clients justifiably want to get on with resolving their problems and issues; therapists often feel pressure to ensure that they have conducted a thorough evaluation and have confidence that the OPIs identified can be substantiated with objective data. This urge on the therapist's part relates to problem analysis or the use of further assessment techniques to understand the root causes of the problem, how it affects the client, the context in which it exists, and its consequences (Pollock & McColl, 1998). Using the OPPM, Stage 3 represents movement from the identification of general OPIs to identification of the specific underlying components or conditions that contribute to the OPIs. In other words, we are moving from the "big picture" to the specific colors and textures that contribute to the painting. The therapist and client must both "buy into" this process and continually collaborate to ensure there is an appropriate balance between evaluation and intervention in the time they spend together. Nothing is more frustrating for both parties than to have spent all of their time on assessment and problem identification, only to have circumstances prevent them from moving on to implementation of intervention strategies. This may result in clearly documented and supported OPIs, but no successful outcomes are achieved because the process was disrupted prior to intervention. For example, consider the habit of using a routine or standard battery of tests on every client who walks through the door. In addition to missing the client-centered boat, the potential problem here is that the test battery may evaluate many occupational performance components, without necessarily identifying issues at the more meaningful level of occupational performance. Proponents of this assessment process may argue it gives them a good picture of the client's skills. However, when tests are administered without a specific, client-identified OPI in mind, much of the information gathered is not used for any purpose, and the assessment can be a waste of time for both the client and the therapist. Client-centered practice is directed by the client's OPIs, not the therapist's test kit.

There is a recurrent ebb and flow throughout the stages of practice, rather than a strictly linear progression from one stage to the next. The occupational therapist may (and probably should in complex cases) come back to Stage 3 after implementing an intervention plan, for further data collection and to refine the approach to intervention. It is also possible to back up one more stage to select a different theoretical framework leading to an alternative assessment approach, subsequently revising the list of factors contributing to the client's OPIs. It is unlikely that there is a clearly marked finish line for each step in the process; it is more like a seamless process of continuous consultation with the client to identify, clarify, and resolve issues limiting occupational performance.

IDENTIFICATION OF PERFORMANCE COMPONENTS AND ENVIRONMENT CONDITIONS

Identifying performance components is the process of observing or measuring skills the client possesses, such as emotional, perceptual, or motor skills (see Table 5-1). Measuring joint range of motion, visual perception, balance, and coordination are examples of ways to identify strengths and limitations in a client's performance components. Identifying environmental conditions is the process of observing the supports and limitations in the environment in which the client functions, including the physical, social, cultural, and institutional environment. Using the Safety Assessment of Function and the Environment for Rehabilitation (SAFER) tool (Oliver, Blathwayt, Brackley, & Tamaki, 1993) is an example of one way to identify environmental conditions specific to a client's home and the interaction between the client's performance and home environment. While assessment tools typically focus on either performance components or environmental conditions, often it is the interaction between the two (the person-environment fit, or misfit) that gives rise to OPIs. (See Law, Cooper, Strong, Stewart, Rigby, & Letts, 1996, for further discussion of the Person-Environment-Occupation interaction.) Providing an inventory of tools for identifying performance components and environmental conditions is beyond the scope of this chapter. Readers are referred to the resources listed at the end of this chapter as a guide to finding relevant assessment tools.

Clearly, it does not make sense to assess all possible performance components in each and every client, as well as all aspects of their physical, social, and cultural environments. How does one decide which components and conditions merit further investigation and, more specifically, which assessment tools to use? The initial interview and process of identifying OPIs provides a range of cues. These cues are either pursued or set aside, based on the pattern in which they present themselves. The combination of issues identified by the client, the therapist's observation of skills and deficits, the age or developmental level of the client, and obvious environmental factors present a picture of the client in context. Patterns may be recognized by the therapist as similar to those presented by past clients, and the process over time requires less effort and becomes more intuitive.

AN EXAMPLE: MEET BOB

The following scenario is based on a case file from community occupational therapy practice. Read Bob's story and select the cues that suggest potential components or conditions contributing to Bob's OPI, which may assist in choosing appropriate assessment tools. It is easier to identify relevant cues if you have a clear goal in mind, relevant to the client's idea of what a successful outcome solution might look like. The client-centered practitioner uses the initial OPI to help decide which cues to pursue or set aside.

Bob says: "I used to spend a lot of my free time reading. Since my stroke, I am unable to read. I can read large printing but it is very slow. I can't always remember what I have read. I want to be able to read books and articles for enjoyment."

Bob's wife had tried bringing him large print books from the library but none of these books held his interest. Taped books had been used but he was not satisfied with these either. The occupational therapist noted that Bob's bookshelves at home were filled with books on history, philosophy, and art.

Bob is a 57-year-old man who sustained a left intrathalamic hemorrhage resulting in dense right hemiplegia, global aphasia, and right hemianopsia. Three months following his stroke, he was discharged from a rehabilitation unit, and it was noted that he showed some improvement in his communication skills, but according to his medical record, the "prognosis remains guarded due to the severity of his impairments." Apraxia and perceptual deficits were considered the major barriers to further functional recovery. It is now 18 months post-stroke, and Bob demonstrates a marked improvement in all areas of his daily function. He is able to speak slowly but clearly, is able to dress and wash himself with less inattention to his right side, and is no longer using a wheelchair to get around.

Questions to ask yourself to help illuminate some of the issues preventing the occupational performance include those listed in Table 5-2. Consider this an exercise in reflective practice, and think about other clients and the internal dialogue you may have with yourself to identify the limitations underlying occupational performance difficulties. The cues in Bob's example are largely performance-based and relate to his potential perceptual deficits; other clients may give cues that would suggest the need for further investigation into environmental conditions. The theoretical approach selected earlier together with the cues identified within the client's story guide the selection of initial tests and measures to identify both the performance components and the environmental conditions that result in difficulties with occupational performance.

Often, we subject clients to the same test over again without thinking about how the client perceives the repetition. An interesting story was presented to the second author from a new therapist working on an acute neurology unit. It was expected that the therapist ask the client orientation questions regarding time and day, and following the therapist's question, the client asked "Doesn't anyone around here have a watch or a calendar? You're the 15th person today who has asked me that question!" This client was obviously feeling frustrated with the repetition and perhaps did not understand the purpose of being asked these questions repetitively. The therapist also noted that many tests had been repeated on the same client and had been reported in the chart by many disciplines, each one with similar results. This situation is avoided when occupational therapists and clients develop a partnership that is client-centered and client-driven. Using this approach, the client has the opportunity to say "You don't need to assess my orientation today; three other people already have, and it's okay." The occupational therapist and client investigate together and decide what needs to be evaluated in order to resolve the issues of importance to the client. This is not intended to suggest that the occupational therapist not share his or her expertise; rather, it is a reminder to listen to the client's story and let it guide the therapist-client interactions. In fact, the therapist must indicate what options are available and work with the client to set a plan in action.

Table 5-2
Thinking Through Factors Contributing to Bob's OPIs

Question	Reflections and Suggestions
What is preventing Bob's ability to read?	Pull the whole picture of the person together by using knowledge of medical conditions, something that the client has identified, or past experiences with other clients. Think about the cognitive and perceptual implications of a CVA and those that were noted by the rehabilitation facility early on in his therapy. Think about the skills required to perform this occupation (reading).
What areas may make the biggest impact for someone with a CVA when trying to read?	It may not be necessary to test every area if we focus on the main skills required for reading and specifically assess those skills.
Are Bob's current visual and perceptual deficits still too severe, thereby making the goal of reading for leisure unreasonable?	It might be preferable to propose to Bob that a quick and simple assessment be done first to determine the answer to this question before proceeding with a comprehensive and possibly time-consuming battery of tests, which may frustrate Bob if they exceed his current skill level.
Do I have the skills and resources to adequately test the components? Are others involved in treatment, and have they previously assessed these performance components?	Ask Bob who else he is working with, what's been tested so far. Discuss options for further evaluation. If you don't have the necessary skills, consider a referral to another occupational therapist with specialized skills in assessing the areas of question or other appropriate disciplines. Also ensure that someone else has not already done the same assessment.
Does Bob understand the purpose of the test, and is he willing to participate? Is the test at the right level for his current abilities (i.e., not too easy or too difficult)?	While it is recognized that the purpose of assessment is to identify Bob's precise skill level, preliminary discussion and observations are used to select tests that will be presented to Bob as available options for learning more about his skill level. Discuss why, what, when, where, and under what conditions the assessments will take place. How the test will assist in planning treatment intervention may also be discussed at this point. Bob should feel comfortable that the assessment plan will enable him to achieve his goal of reading. This negotiation is fundamental to informed consent and decision-making on Bob's part.

Table 5-2 (continued) **Thinking Through Factors Contributing to Bob's OPIs**	
Question	Reflections and Suggestions
When will I have enough information to begin discussion of goals and treatment options? Will I need this information now, or can I collect more later?	Most therapists are limited with respect to the time allowed with each client, whether it is due to caseload, financial influences, or time allotted to each client for participation in a program. Assessment must be tailored to meet the needs of the client and the program; sufficient information must be gathered without "overassessing." Decide how much information is required now, to guide actions and decisions in the immediate future. You can always come back to assessment, if required, at any point in the OPPM loop.
What additional information do I need to make an intervention decision?	Perhaps a perceptual-cognitive theoretical framework offers some suggestions for assessment. The assessment results may be used to refine Bob's original OPI (or perhaps to broaden it to include additional occupations affected by the same performance components), and these results can be discussed with Bob to set targeted outcomes and plan interventions. (Targeted outcomes and interventions are the subjects of subsequent chapters.)
Remember the "client as expert," and reflect back to selected cues for validation by the client.	For example, why were previous interventions, such as large-print books and books on tape, not satisfactory to Bob?

FORMAL VS. INFORMAL ASSESSMENT TOOLS

Armed with a list of priority OPIs and a collection of cues that suggest the performance components and environmental conditions that require assessment, the therapist needs to select appropriate tools. Assessments may be either informal (relatively unstructured) or formal (such as standardized tests and measures). Informal assessments make use of observation, trial and error, and common sense in order to make judgments about a client's performance. They may be used when only a quick observation of a skill is necessary (e.g., toilet transfers), or for performance areas for which customized observation rather than a standardized protocol is deemed more appropriate. For example, if the client identifies a very specific OPI, such as difficulty making tea, it may make more sense to informally observe her making tea in her own kitchen. The occupational therapist observes component skills and environmental assets and liabilities in order to make subsequent suggestions to address the OPI. Trial and error may be used, such as "try lifting the kettle this way" when problems are noted, and the result of alternate methods can also be observed. This may, in some instances, be preferable to a complete standardized assessment of cooking skills, which may be out of proportion to the stated OPI, too long, or designed for an entirely different client population and therefore can't be accurately interpreted for this specific client.

The credibility of informal approaches may be enhanced by ensuring that observations are made objectively and have meaning to the individual client. If both the client and the therapist can agree on an objective description of the target behavior, and identify what improvement would look like, then this might be a suitable method of assessing performance components or environmental conditions in that context. An example: The client wants to be able to pour a glass of milk from a brand new 2-liter (2-quart) carton of milk. Limitations in hand strength and coordination are contributing factors, but a standardized grip strength measurement has little meaning to the client in this situation—what's important is achieving the task. The therapist and client can objectively measure hand strength by using the task of pouring milk as the measurement tool. It can be used both to identify the limitation in hand strength and to measure improvement after a period of intervention. Credibility is enhanced by documenting precisely what success looks like (e.g., lifting the carton with one hand, pouring the milk into a glass without spilling). Provided that both client and therapist can reach agreement on the criteria for success, the need for sophisticated or more complex assessment is not always necessary. Single subject research designs are great sources of information on documenting a functionally relevant outcome measure for individual clients.

Standardized tests and measures are those tools that have published protocols, with specific instructions for administering the test. Typically, they will report evidence of reliability and validity with one or more client populations and, if appropriate to the type of test, normative data that indicate the expected performance. Even if a test manual states it is reliable with a specific population, it is wise to assess this yourself in your own setting. A quick interrater or test-retest reliability check will help ensure that standardized instructions are being adhered to and that the test is reliable with representatives from your own client group. Some examples of "best practice" in the tests available for measuring occupational performance areas are documented in a textbook edited by Law, Baum, and Dunn (2000).

Things to think about when selecting standardized tests and measures or evaluating a new test include the following:

- **Purpose of the test.** What performance components or environmental conditions will this test measure? For what client populations (age group, diagnostic group) is it appropriate? What theoretical approach underlies this test?

- **Clinical utility.** Will it be useful? Does it provide a "just right challenge" for my clients? How long does it take to administer, to score, to learn to use it? How much does it cost? Are there any practical limitations? For example, a home care therapist can hardly cart around dozens of tests in the back seat of her car. Tests that are expensive per use, used rarely, and use equipment not easily transported are readily eliminated from her repertoire.

- **Reliability.** Is the test consistent? If someone else administers the test, will we get the same result (interrater reliability)? If I administer the test on two different occasions, to a client whose status has not changed, will I get the same result (test-retest reliability)? Is it reliable with clients who have similar characteristics to my clients?
- **Validity.** Do the results say something about the skills the test is intended to measure? For example, does a test of hand function really measure how people use their hands? Further, when practicing from the perspective of occupational performance and client-centered practice, a test of hand function would ideally tell you more than just the level of hand strength or dexterity. A valid test would also help link the performance component (hand strength, dexterity) to how that level of performance impacts on the way clients use their hands to do daily occupations (closer to the level of stated OPIs).
- **Responsiveness.** Is the test responsive to change in client status? For example, when a client's mental status changes, is this accurately reflected by a changed "score" on the test used? This is essential if you intend to use the test to monitor client progress.

Some of the advantages and limitations of formal vs. informal assessment are indicated in Table 5-3.

It is important to remember that using assessments to enhance a one-to-one client-therapist partnership designed to resolve client-specified OPIs is quite different than measuring occupational performance status in a research project or collecting data for program evaluation purposes. The intended audience will influence the selection of assessment approaches to a certain degree. Identify who the audience is and what they value. Does this assessment need to make sense to the client alone, or does it also need to include ways to measure the success of the rehabilitation program? Combining methods or supplementing the method that is most relevant to the client with tools that meet agency requirements for program evaluation or total quality management may be a reasonable approach. For example, if the client's only OPI under the occupational performance area of self-care is inability to wash her hair, but the program in which she is a client requires a specific activities of daily living tool to be completed in order to measure program outcomes, it may be feasible to integrate the two approaches and meet the needs of all parties. Make use of whatever is contained in a "required outcome data set," but also think critically from the perspective of the client's OPIs and use this to guide assessment choices.

A different way to categorize assessment approaches is as qualitative and quantitative approaches. Many of the standardized assessment tools would fall into a quantitative approach, because they seek to measure or quantify performance. However, qualitative approaches also provide useful data and can also be both informal and more rigorous in application. At the less formal end of the continuum, a qualitative approach would seek to understand the client's perspective regarding a specific OPI, perhaps by using narrative (i.e., asking the client to describe or tell a story about the OPI). More formal qualitative approaches would implement processes described in grounded theory or ethnographic research and are generally too labor intensive for routine clinical practice.

A final issue deals with proxy reporting. When a client cannot communicate, or when circumstances suggest that there are "associate clients" such as parents, spouses, or other

---

Table 5-3
Advantages and Limitations of
Standardized and Informal Assessments

Standardized (Formal)
Advantages
- Once procedures are learned, it becomes easier and routine and you know the data it will generate.
- Once educated, others (e.g., team members) understand the data and results.
- Can compare client to others (e.g., judge "how able" a client is relative to others in similar situations).
- May document progress.

Limitations
- Standard equipment and materials may be unwieldy to cart around.
- May be expensive to own several tests.
- May need special training to administer and score.
- Client may not match the population for which the test was standardized.
- May seem contrived or unsuitable in some circumstances or for some clients.
- May require assessing a much broader range of skills than is necessary to investigate the client's OPI.
- The urge to "wing it" or change the test invalidates the results.

Informal (Non-Standardized)
Advantages
- Customized to client's skill level, needs, and interests (very client-centered).
- May be quick and to the point.
- Makes use of what's readily available, no specialized equipment, relies on observation.

Limitations
- Therapist must be quick-witted, able to "think on his or her feet" to come up with suitable tasks (sometimes).
- Can't easily (mathematically) make comparisons across clients.
- More difficult to replicate (without specified procedures); therefore, may not accurately measure change or progress.
- Has questionable credibility for some purposes.

---

caregivers, much of the preceding assessment will involve a proxy. To whatever extent it is possible to validate findings with the primary client, this should be done. Assessment of environmental conditions may involve others even when a client is fully able to participate in the assessment process. For example, a child's teacher or a worker's immediate supervisor may often provide useful information about the productivity demands within the client's environment, when school- or work-related OPIs have been identified.

ANALYSIS OF FINDINGS

Once data on performance components and environmental conditions have been collected, it is time to link the information back to the original OPIs, discuss the findings with the client, and determine how the client wishes to proceed.

Data are analyzed following the assessment to ensure primary causes of occupational performance dysfunction are clearly understood. What was previously a suspected component or condition influencing performance is now confirmed or refuted. The therapist may find similar causes of dysfunction underlying different OPIs (e.g., limitations in strength and endurance may contribute to difficulties with performing work-related tasks, keeping up with housecleaning, and active leisure pursuits, all of which were stated OPIs for a particular client). Discussing the assessment results with the client may lead to a wish to revise the OPIs based on new insight gained from the results. Clients may have greater comfort in discussing the direction they want therapy to take once they have a clear idea of the limitations underlying their original OPIs. The client may have additional insights and be able to give the therapist an indication of agreement with the apparent cause of dysfunction, or suggest whether there are more complex factors interacting with the cause or whether he or she feels the cause is significant to the OPI. The crucial aspect of analysis is to identify which performance components and environmental conditions should be targeted for action (Townsend et al., 1997).

After discussing results with the client, reflect on all of the available information. Do the new data make sense within the theoretical approach that was selected earlier, (i.e., is the selected theory still compatible with the results)? How will these data be used to proceed to the next step in the process? Is there sufficient information to guide subsequent stages in the OPPM (setting outcomes, selecting interventions)? The therapist continues collaborating with the client and explains how information can be used to continue the process of determining available resources, negotiating targeted outcomes, and discussing potential action plans.

CONCLUSION

The importance of continuous therapist-client collaboration cannot be overemphasized if the assessment process is to be worthwhile in identifying performance components and environmental conditions contributing to the client's priority OPIs. There is constant interaction throughout the process between client and therapist through negotiation, explanation, and clarification. The therapist, in addition to listening to the client's ideas of some of the potential inhibitors of performance, also uses theory to analyze potential causes including performance and environmental factors. At this point, therapists draw on their experience and use clinical reasoning and intuition to help put together the pieces of the puzzle. The therapist is advised to use the client's OPIs as an indicator of eventual goals, recognize important cues that suggest the most appropriate methods of observing or measuring performance, explain the reasons for testing specific areas to the client, and try to avoid subjecting clients to unnecessary tests or overassessment.

Applying theoretical knowledge (Chapter 4) helps uncover the cause of occupational performance dysfunction. The client brings the issues to the table and usually has a good idea of some of the contributing factors and the desired therapy outcome. Clients may need assistance in identifying specific causes and working through the steps to get where they want to go. Careful attention to the client's most important issues and working collaboratively with the client throughout the assessment process will lead to a more satisfying outcome. Respect the client's expertise in problem identification, and share theoretical knowledge and past experiences to help guide the selection of efficient assessment methods. Negotiate the assessment plan using language that the client understands to ensure informed decision-making can occur. Results of both formal and informal assessment guide ongoing discussions with clients, providing a basis for explanation of potential causes of dysfunction and possible strategies for resolving issues. This discussion is crucial when negotiating targeted outcomes and developing action plans.

Remember the department store shopper who went looking for new carpet and was almost sold a sofa. Resist the urge to be the know-it-all salesperson. Instead, be the attentive sales consultant. Listen to the client's story, offer suggestions, and engage in a dialogue aimed at identifying the client's OPIs and the underlying causes of those issues. In the long run, the client-centered approach is more likely to achieve meaningful and satisfactory outcomes than other approaches that fail to identify the client's perspective on goals for therapy.

RESOURCES FOR OCCUPATIONAL THERAPY ASSESSMENT, TESTS, AND MEASURES

American Occupational Therapy Foundation. OT Assessments web page. <http://www.aotf.org/html/ot_assessments.html> This page, within the American Occupational Therapy Foundation's web site, is a database of occupational therapy assessments indexed in OT Bibsys (Occupational Therapy Bibliographic System). Assessment tools can be searched by keyword, title, or author.

Asher, I.E. (1996). *Occupational therapy assessment tools: An annotated index.* (2nd ed.). Bethesda, MD: American Occupational Therapy Association, Inc. Each test cited in this book is summarized with a brief description of the purpose, clientele, administration, psychometric properties, and source for test kits, manuals, or instructions.

Kielhofner, G., Mallinson, T., & de las Heras, C.G. (1995). Methods of data gathering. In G. Kielhofner (Ed.), *A Model of Human Occupation: Theory and Application* (2nd ed., pp. 205-250). Baltimore, MD: Williams & Wilkins. Suggestions for gathering data regarding client performance.

Law, M.C., Baum, C.M., & Dunn, W. (2000). *Measuring occupational performance: A guide to best practice.* Thorofare, NJ: SLACK Incorporated. Contains suggestions for ways of assessing occupational performance areas and performance components, including reviews of "best" available measurement tools.

Law, M., King, G., MacKinnon, E., Russell, D., Murphy, C., Hurley, P., & Bosch, E. (1999). *All about outcomes: An educational program to help you understand, evaluate, and choose pediatric outcome measures* [CD-ROM]. Thorofare, NJ: SLACK Incorporated. An interactive software program to guide in the selection of appropriate measures from more than 135 pediatric outcomes measures.

Reed, K.L. (1991). *Quick reference to occupational therapy.* Gaithersburg, MD: Aspen. Helpful listings under specific disorders of component areas and assessments to consider. Also provides an appendix of references for specific occupational therapy tests.

REFERENCES

Canadian Association of Occupational Therapists (CAOT) (1991). *Occupational therapy guidelines for client-centred practice.* Toronto, Ontario, Canada: CAOT Publications ACE.

Fearing, V.G., Law, M., & Clark, J. (1997). An occupational performance process model: Fostering client and therapist alliances. *Canadian Journal of Occupational Therapy, 64,* 7-15.

Law, M.C., Baum, C.M., & Dunn, W. (2000). *Measuring occupational performance: A guide to best practice.* Thorofare, NJ: SLACK Incorporated.

Law, M., Cooper, B., Strong, S., Stewart, D., Rigby, P., & Letts, L. (1996). The Person-Environment-Occupation model: A transactive approach to occupational performance. *Canadian Journal of Occupational Therapy, 63,* 9-23.

Oliver, R., Blathwayt, J., Brackley, C., & Tamaki, T. (1993). Development of the Safety Assessment of Function and the Environment for Rehabilitation (SAFER) tool. *Canadian Journal of Occupational Therapy, 60,* 78-82.

Pollock, N., & McColl, M.A. (1998). Assessment in client-centred occupational therapy. In M. Law (Ed.), *Client-Centered Occupational Therapy.* Thorofare, NJ: SLACK Incorporated.

Townsend, E., Stanton, S., Law, M., Polatajko, H., Baptiste, S., Thompson-Franson, T., Kramer, C., Swedlove, F., Brintnell, S., & Campanile, L. (1997). *Enabling occupation: An occupational therapy perspective.* Ottawa, Ontario, Canada: CAOT Publications.

chapter six

Stage 4

NAMING STRENGTHS AND RESOURCES OF THE CLIENT AND THE THERAPIST

SANDRA HALE, BSc, OT(C)

A SHIFT IN EMPHASIS

In the fourth stage of the Occupational Performance Process Model (OPPM) (Fearing, Law, & Clark, 1997), the therapist and client collaboratively determine strengths and resources to be woven into the therapy process. Previous stages have illuminated occupational performance issues (OPIs), theoretical approaches, performance components, and environmental conditions contributing to issues (Chapters 3 through 5). Strengths and resources revealed during the narration, which began in Stage 1, are validated at this time. The identification of issues can be paired with available strengths and resources to enhance performance in issue areas. At the same time, therapists identify and integrate their own strengths and resources to work in the most effective way with clients.

There is little evidence in the literature that therapists ensure strengths and resources are identified and incorporated in the occupational therapy process. Rather, some literature suggests this step may be omitted, at times to the detriment of the therapeutic outcome (Carlson, 1996; Corring & Cook, 1999; Price-Lackey & Cashman, 1996; Sherr-Klein, 1997; Stoch, 1999). The ability to see possibilities within even devastating injury or illness is an aspect of hope (Spencer, Davidson, & White, 1997). Ensuring client strengths and resources are identified and incorporated into therapy can foster hope in the process of recovery.

STRENGTHS AND RESOURCES: ENHANCING INTERVENTION

Using the Person-Environment-Occupation (PEO) model (Law, Cooper, Strong, Stewart, Rigby, & Letts, 1996) as a framework to determine strengths and resources assists in conceptualizing this stage of the process model. Strengths are found within the person, resources are found in environments, and both are found in occupation. The PEO model is represented by three concentric circles interacting dynamically (Law et al., 1996; Strong, Rigby, Stewart, Law, Letts, & Cooper, 1999). The identification of strengths and resources is also dynamic. As a client engages in therapy, different strengths may be recognized and capitalized upon. Recognition and integration of personal, environmental, and occupational strengths and resources may happen throughout the process loop. Once a strength is identified, it can be used to help address an OPI.

For example, a client experiencing repeated depressive episodes identifies an issue of diminished ability to parent his children when depressed. With further dialogue, he identifies putting the children to bed and reading to them in a manner he used to enjoy as a priority issue. He also identifies a personal strength in his creativity. He states he used to be accomplished in creative writing and would like to try this activity again. During occupational therapy, while in the hospital, he writes a short story complete with pictures on the computer. He returns to the hospital after a weekend at home and reports he read the book to his children. This provided a sense of accomplishment in his ability to engage in parenting activities. By pairing an identified strength (creativity) with an identified issue (diminished ability to read to his children), his occupational performance was enhanced.

CLIENT STRENGTHS AND RESOURCES: THE HOW TO'S

Identification of strengths and resources may be elicited through the use of guided questions and exploring client narratives. The following section is separated into the three spheres of the PEO model. Potential questions that could be incorporated into already available assessments are located at the end of each section. It is not intended that these questions be used in their entirety with each client, nor is it an exhaustive list. Questions should be guided according to the uniqueness of each client and situation.

CLIENT STRENGTHS IN PERSON

Personal strengths might include attributes, abilities, inner resources, values, and beliefs, both spiritual and cultural. Determining personal strengths requires that we know the inner resources and capabilities of the person. Clients often articulate these through narration and demonstrate them by what they do in a variety of situations. Strengths in the person category may be identified by significant people in the client's life, particularly if the client is unable to participate fully in this process.

Mike Hawkes sustained an incomplete spinal cord injury while playing hockey and spent months in rehabilitation. He describes the importance of recognizing personal strengths.

During the first 2 months of my injury, my body was paralyzed from the nipple line down, with no use of my arms and hands. The ability to get to know me was as important as any medication the medical staff was putting into my body. Both therapists (occupational and physical therapist) spent the time to understand me, mean-

ing they asked questions of my "former life," which identified my personality type and the activities I pursued. They learned I was a classic type A personality: a hard worker and one who engaged in almost every sport known to man. They recognized they did not have a quitter and accommodated my desire to use more of my off time doing the rehab exercises they had taught during my session times. M. Hawkes (personal communication, May 10, 1999)

In Stages 1 and 4, listening to client narrative provides the opportunity to know the person beyond his or her current situation. When clients experience significant change in their ability, recognizing personal strengths can assist in developing new strategies and incorporating previously used strategies to resolve issues. The identification of personal strengths may help clients recognize that they remain the essence of who they have always been, despite loss of function. This is described by Cashman "...and I discovered that ... who I was as a core person wasn't lost and wasn't damaged" (Price-Lackey & Cashman, 1996, p. 311).

Questions to Promote Reflection on Personal Strengths
- What do you consider to be your personal strengths?
- If I were to ask your best friend or someone who knows you well, how might they describe you?
- Can you think of someone whom you have valued and respected and why?
- What has helped you get through difficult situations in the past?
- What do you value most?
- Do you have a belief, faith, or spiritual guidance that gives you strength?
- What is most significant in your life?

CLIENT RESOURCES IN ENVIRONMENT

The Canadian Model of Occupational Performance defines environment to include cultural, institutional, physical, and social components (Canadian Association of Occupational Therapists [CAOT], 1997). This broadened perspective of environment assists occupational therapists to examine the resources many clients have. Environments are as unique as the individuals in them.

There is a tendency in occupational therapy to focus on the "doing" (Wilcock, 1998). We may move too quickly to "do" interventions that are known and commonly used to resolve issues. Collaborating with clients to identify potential resources may provide unique opportunities for resolving performance issues.

For example, if a client identifies difficulty feeding or dressing him- or herself due to physical limitations, a therapist might consider an adaptive aid or technique to promote independence with this activity. In some cultures, however, it may be normal and possibly expected that a friend or family member perform tasks such as these for someone who has difficulty doing so. Without exploring resources available to individual clients within the context of a personal environment, interventions that have little meaning could be suggested and a potential resolution missed. Although this may be a different perspective on independence than the therapist might have, using a cultural or social resource rather than an adaptive aid may resolve an issue for a client and be perfectly satisfactory to him or her. In fact, it may add an aspect of pleasure to both parties and allow for further pursuit of occupations, which are more important to the client.

Exploring client environments for resources may reveal available services. It includes looking at community and financial resources, work, home, society, and health care environments, including the people within these. Community centers, libraries, shopping centers, grocery stores, volunteer associations, and senior centers often offer services that can be used by clients. In all four realms of environment (cultural, social, physical, and institutional) (CAOT, 1997), there are possibilities. As overwhelming as this may sound, pairing resources with client-driven issues should provide for more satisfactory outcomes and, in the end, save time.

Questions to Promote Reflection on Potential Resources in the Client's Environment

Social
- Who are the people in your life who are most important to you?
- Would it be helpful or feasible to have them involved in some of the things we might do together?
- How could I as a therapist be a resource to you?

Physical
- What could you use within your home that would be helpful to you? Examples may include equipment that is useful, places that provide comfort, areas that enable you to perform daily tasks.
- Within your workplace, what is or might be helpful to you?

Institutional
- Are there services available that you have used to assist you in the past?
- Are you aware of how you might access financial resources in order to address issues you have identified?

Cultural
- Do you have beliefs or routines that you particularly value?

CLIENT STRENGTHS AND RESOURCES IN OCCUPATION

Occupational strengths are past, present, and future occupations that represent important roles and achievements to the person. They define and provide meaning to daily lives and promote health (Law et al., 1996; Wilcock, 1998). Identifying occupational strengths demonstrates clients are valued as people and their abilities, in whatever state they may be, are important. Occupational strengths are the interplay of personal strengths and environmental resources that enable clients to perform meaningful tasks.

The following continues Mike's story with his view of using strengths in person, resources in environment, and the promotion of occupational performance based on his occupational strengths.

I had been an avid swimmer before my injury, and, in learning of the avail-ability of a pool, the occupational and physical therapists enabled my desire to par-ticipate in this activity by altering therapy times. Additionally, both therapists engaged me as a role model to other patients, allowing me to give of my time. This gave me a sense of purpose in my diminished role as an active person. As well, they identified that as a past police officer I had discipline and could take direction eas-ily and was frustrated when my best efforts were of a failing conclusion. On these occasions, they demonstrated compassion and understanding. M. Hawkes (person-al communication, May 10, 1999)

Questions to Promote Reflection on Client Occupational Strengths and Resources

- What activities have you done at work, school, home, or in your leisure/recreation that you recall with a feeling of pride?
- What have you done in the past that you would not want to give up?
- What roles do you have that are particularly important to you?
- Can you think of a time when things were going well in your life? What were you doing at those times?

An assessment that examines potential losses and gains in occupation with changes in function is the Community Adaptive Planning Assessment (CAPA) recently developed by the CAPA Project Group, School of Occupational Therapy, Texas Woman's University. By focusing on adapting to life change, past experience and strengths are considered in setting occupational goals (Spencer & Davidson, 1998). It provides a framework for eval-uating losses and gains when individuals experience change in function.

WHEN A CLIENT STRUGGLES TO IDENTIFY STRENGTHS AND RESOURCES

The approach used in identifying strengths and resources requires individualization. When clients are struggling, asking them to state their strengths may negatively alter the therapeutic alliance that can develop between therapist and client. When clients have expe-rienced significant change to their physical state, such as paralysis, brain injury, burn, or stroke, this represents a catastrophic event that will permanently alter their lives. Each per-son's acceptance of loss, in the process of his or her recovery, will vary markedly. Clients may wonder what strengths they have left, particularly if they defined personal strengths by phys-ical ability. Clients who experience symptoms of depression, anxiety, or any long-standing issues that have altered their function may also have difficulty identifying strengths. They may have experienced loss in productive roles, socially in their relationships with others, and limitations in their capacity to enjoy recreation, all of which can erode a sense of self-worth. Perhaps family and friends are not sources of support or encouragement; therefore, asking these clients to identify resources may only further identify components or barriers.

Therapists will need to judge what is the best way to identify strengths and resources dictated by the unique needs of the client. Ensuring strengths and resources are woven into therapy assures clients there is purpose in identifying them. Rather than pointedly asking this group of clients what their strengths and resources are, incorporating questions within conversation provides a less formal method of discovering them. The therapist may reflect back to the client strengths and resources observed during various interactions. Some clients may have difficulty naming even one strength or resource. This can be an important statement of where this person is in recovery and how he or she views life at present. A friend or family member may have a different perspective and, therefore, can be helpful in recognition of personal traits and accomplishments.

THERAPIST STRENGTHS AND RESOURCES

THERAPIST STRENGTHS IN PERSON

A therapist's personal strengths may include an ability to develop interpersonal relationships, respect client choices, seek assistance when needed, provide leadership (see Chapter 1), apply extensive skill and knowledge, and commit to life-long learning. All these strengths would assist in realization of the values and beliefs of occupational therapy, as stated in *Enabling Occupation: An Occupational Therapy Perspective* (CAOT, 1997).

Technical care (the application of therapeutic techniques) is believed to be the best information available to pass on to clients. It represents "best practice" to produce greatest improvement in health (Donabedian, 1988). This technical aspect of the therapeutic interaction is important; however, it can be lost if not communicated in a meaningful way to clients. "The interpersonal process is the vehicle by which technical care is implemented and on which its success depends" (Donabedian, 1988, p. 1744). The importance of this interpersonal aspect of care is underrated in current health care trends (Cassidy, 1999). The ability to develop an interpersonal connection to the client is likely to have the most enduring impact.

> *There is no greater gift than to feel listened to, understood, and valued for your opinion. The therapist who had the biggest impact as I was recovering was a real listener; she asked me a lot of questions and also shared parts of her life. If someone listens to me, it breeds a natural respect, and I am more likely to listen to [him or her].*
> W. Lawrence (personal communication, July 29, 1999)

It is not possible to separate ourselves from the therapeutic process. Knowing our strengths and limitations increases our capacity to facilitate a client's process. Recognizing when we are not connecting to clients may be an indication that a critical component of client-centered practice may be missing. (See Chapter 13 for guidelines for evaluating client-centered process.)

Questions to Promote Reflections on Therapist Personal Strengths

- Can I put myself in this client's situation and understand his or her picture of the future?
- Can I move beyond feelings of sympathy to facilitate a therapeutic process mentally, emotionally, and physically for this individual?
- Are there personal issues I am facing that may require attention in order for me to be a more effective therapist with this individual?
- When I work with clients, do I ensure I have heard their narrative and know them as a person before making suggestions for intervention?
- Do I have the skills to complete assessments or interventions required to enhance performance with this individual?

THERAPIST RESOURCES IN ENVIRONMENT

Broadening our view of environment to include cultural, institutional, physical, and social elements means looking at our resources differently. Therapists can support resolution of issues by collaborating with clients to integrate all possible resources effectively. This challenges our profession to ensure environmental resources are conducive to client-centered practice (see Chapter 2).

- **Cultural resources.** Respecting cultural identity may require occupational therapists to have information available in different languages, recognize ceremonial practices as a component of occupational performance, and ensure there is consideration of the spiritual aspect of a person's life.
- **Institutional resources.** Occupational therapists can be advocates for services that suit clients' needs and fit their time frames of recovery. Therapists can act as brokers between institutions and clients. Understanding clients within the contexts of their own environments makes it easier to see what would be a best fit and to determine needed resources. Including clients in decision-making and ensuring individuality is respected can assist clients in developing the skills and confidence to advocate for themselves.
- **Physical resources.** The physical esthetics of our environments affect us. Ensuring equipment and tools used in therapy are current and meaningful to clients and that physical surroundings are inviting can impact occupational performance.
- **Social resources.** Creating atmospheres of respect and openness for client interactions can also enhance performance. Pairing clients with others at different stages of recovery, encouraging socialization with group activities, and creating opportunity to be with others can be part of using social resources to effect change.

The influence of environment on clients' occupational performance may detract or enhance it. Resources allocated according to system guidelines, rather than the unique needs of clients, will often detract and frustrate clients and therapists (Stoch, 1999). Occupational therapists can be instrumental in altering or adding resources in environments to better fit client needs. Identification of resources may highlight gaps, inefficiencies, and need for revising outdated practices. Using the OPPM in clinical practice facilitates greater understanding of what assists clients most. Environments can then be adapted to best suit the individuals.

As health care, community funding, or insurance systems are often unfamiliar to clients and their families, the process of identifying resources within environments assists therapists and clients to understand and access these systems. A therapist can be a resource to clients by being knowledgeable of system resources. In order to recommend resources, therapists must know the person well enough to ensure it fits the client's context. This includes being aware of when best to recommend resources.

Clients who responded to requests for input into this chapter indicated that when recovering from illness or injury, they may not have the energy or desire to utilize all the environmental resources at the time of their rehabilitation. Should this be the case, it may be of more benefit to equip clients with the information or skills needed to access resources at later times. As much as possible, therapists can explore their environment for resources by seeing them firsthand or making phone calls to gather information. Being familiar with resources in the environment ensures therapists are accurate sources of information.

Questions to Promote Reflection on Therapist Resources in Environment
- Do I have the necessary assessment and intervention resources to meet client needs?
- Do I have access to a quiet, private place to see clients?
- Does the environment in which I work as an occupational therapist provide resources that best fit client needs?
- Does the program meet client needs? (See Chapters 9 and 11.)

THERAPIST STRENGTHS AND RESOURCES IN OCCUPATION

As indicated previously, interactions between therapist and client include interpersonal and technical aspects of care. The importance of interpersonal relationships has been highlighted. Equally important is the need for therapists to be competent in occupational therapy practice. The advancement of technology and various medical treatments will affect our occupation. Ongoing restructuring of health care services presents both opportunity and challenge to remain current. Occupation is enhanced by the integration of personal strengths and environmental resources. Taking part in educational opportunities maintains technical expertise. This strengthens our occupation as a therapist.

The profession of occupational therapy is fortunate to have opportunities to venture into a variety of practice domains. When therapists choose to make shifts into different areas of practice, there may be a need to adjust styles to suit certain populations of clients. It may also highlight the need for further learning in a clinical area. Recognizing this need is a personal strength. Accessing the resources to address learning enhances our occupational success.

Questions to Promote Reflection of Therapist Occupational Strengths and Resources
- Am I suited to working in this area of practice or do I find myself struggling?
- Would taking further education or networking with other therapists assist me in this area of practice?
- Is there balance in my occupations of self-care, productivity, and leisure?

INTEGRATING STRENGTHS AND RESOURCES INTO INTERVENTION: PARTNERING WITH CLIENTS

Identifying issues in the first stages of the process model could create an overall vision of disability or a focus on that which is not working, without the balance of Stage 4. Although identification of issues elucidates our reason for working with clients, to **partner** with them broadens the potential scope of the therapeutic relationship. Partnership can be a method of rapport building, empowerment, recognition of ability, and a process of discovery. Without it, opportunities may potentially be missed. As with all other stages of the OPPM, it is considered to be an integral aspect of client-centered practice (Fearing et al., 1997).

Partnering with clients requires a complex set of interpersonal and technical skills. Clients' strengths may be camouflaged traits often judged by others in a negative light. Yet these may be the very elements to capitalize upon in therapy. For example, the "unrealistic" may be dreamers, the "difficult" determined, the "noncompliant" independent, the "unmotivated" not yet challenged. By identifying strengths and resources, choices in intervention will reflect our collaborative efforts with clients. Offering choice is not client-centered practice, but respecting choice is. Informing clients of our perspective in a partnership should assist them to make decisions that fit their circumstances and preferences. This requires occupational therapists to be knowledgeable of clients' abilities despite their illness or injury and to be sensitive to the emotional process a client may be in.

Occupational therapists value inclusion of client perspectives as reflected in current models of practice (CAOT, 1997). Assessments, written documentation, and literature that demonstrate the consideration of client and therapist strengths and resources are presently sparse. Ensuring inclusion will enhance our relationships with clients and allow us to combine our resources and strengths so that better outcomes can be achieved.

ACKNOWLEDGMENTS

I would like to thank all the people who graciously gave their time to tell the story of their experiences with rehabilitation, which assisted in the writing of this chapter.

REFERENCES

Canadian Association of Occupational Therapists (CAOT) (1997). *Enabling occupation: An occupational therapy perspective*. Ottawa, Ontario, Canada: CAOT Publications ACE.

Carlson, J. (1996). Evaluating patient motivation in physical disabilities practice settings. *American Journal of Occupational Therapy, 51*, 347-351.

Cassidy, D. (1999). Measuring outcomes. *Recovery, 10*, 15-17.

Corring, D., & Cook, J. (1999). Client-centred care means that I am a valued human being. *Canadian Journal of Occupational Therapy, 66*, 71-82.

Donabedian, A. (1988). The quality of care: How can it be assessed? *Journal of the American Medical Association, 260*, 1743-1748.

Fearing, V.G., Law, M., & Clark, J. (1997). An occupational performance process model: Fostering client and therapist alliances. *Canadian Journal of Occupational Therapy, 64*, 7-15.

Law, M., Cooper, B., Strong, S., Stewart, D., Rigby, P., & Letts, L. (1996). The Person-Environment-Occupation model: A transactive approach to occupational performance. *Canadian Journal of Occupational Therapy, 63*, 9-23.

Price-Lackey, P., & Cashman, J. (1996). Jenny's story: Reinventing oneself through occupation and narrative configuration. *American Journal of Occupational Therapy, 50*, 306-314.

Sherr-Klein, B. (1997). *Slow dance: A story of stroke, love and disability.* Toronto, Ontario, Canada: Random House.

Spencer, J., & Davidson, H. (1998). The Community Adaptive Planning Assessment: A clinical tool for documenting future planning with clients. *American Journal of Occupational Therapy, 52*, 19-30.

Spencer, J., Davidson, H., & White, V. (1997). Helping clients develop hopes for the future. *American Journal of Occupational Therapy, 51*, 191-198.

Stoch, D. (1999). Identifying the client: The challenge of client-centred practice in a fee-for-service system. *Occupational Therapy Now, March/April*, 8-9.

Strong, S., Rigby, P., Stewart D., Law, M., Letts, L., & Cooper, B. (1999). Application of the Person-Environment-Occupation model: A practical tool. *Canadian Journal of Occupational Therapy, 66*, 122-133.

Wilcock, A.A. (1998). Reflections on doing, being and becoming. *Canadian Journal of Occupational Therapy, 65*, 248-256.

chapter seven

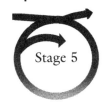

Stage 5

Collaborating on Targeted Outcomes and Making Action Plans

Jo Clark, BSc(OT), OT(C), Brian Bell

Stages 1 through 4 of the Occupational Performance Process Model (OPPM) (naming, validating, and prioritizing occupational performance issues [OPIs]; selecting potential intervention models; identifying occupational performance components and conditions; and identifying strengths and resources) constitute the data-gathering phases of the "loop" (Fearing, Law, & Clark, 1997). In Stage 5, the question now becomes what do we do about the issues and the contributing factors presented? Historically, therapists have felt that developing the plan fell into their domain of expertise. Often, the therapeutic relationship begins as a collaborative process with the therapist and client gathering information together. If, however, the therapist takes this information away to plan from, the relationship is now one-sided as intervention evolves from this "outline." At times, professionals may need to organize their thoughts in terms of what they may be able to offer by way of intervention. However, this should be thought of as a draft that can be brought back to the client for further input. Together they can shape this outline into a cohesive plan based on mutual understanding. When they don't plan together, there is potential for division, and the process may grind to a halt. While making use of the therapist's knowledge base and clinical reasoning is important, doing so in the absence of client direction and participation has obvious outcomes of frustration for both parties. In such a structure, clients lack presence as unique individuals, and therapy moves in a direction that is driven more by therapist or program goals than those of the individual client.

The authors formed a partnership to write this chapter as it is based in something we feel passionate about…**believing**. This connection between believers was initiated when Jo interviewed Brian using the Canadian Occupational Performance Measure (COPM) (Law, Baptiste, Carswell, McColl, Polatajko, & Pollock, 1998). Reflecting our belief that in the occupational therapy process both client and therapist have a voice, in this chapter, authors' voices will be identified throughout. Brian's name will precede his narration giving insight to the client's perspective. Jo's voice will connect us to current occupational therapy practice with all the segments in between. The process of authorship was one in which we both truly learned from each other, collaboration in the merging of beliefs and experiences.

Brian: Prior to this kind of narrative style of interaction between client and therapist, I had been asked by an occupational therapist what I needed. My response was that I didn't know. I had never been a quadriplegic before. I was frequently approached with the idea of learning to dress or brush my teeth, while tales of my previous life in the outdoors seemed to fall by the wayside as unnecessary information. During this storytelling style of interview (COPM), I felt listened to and believed in. The connection was so strong that I spoke of future desires with comfort and was neither discredited nor discouraged as having false hope. Although I have a long journey ahead, I feel empowered in the fact that some hear and some believe.

Through the COPM and subsequent meetings, Jo formed a vision of Brian in context.
Who is Brian Bell?
- He is a storyteller and philosopher.
- He is Kirsten's partner.
- He is a spirit and soul of gargantuan proportion.
- He is the infant that rocked his crib across the room and against the door.
- He is Stephanie's and Keeley's dad.
- He is a lover of nature, a mountain cyclist, a skier, a swimmer, and scuba diver.
- He is the son of Alec and Cathy, and brother to Tracie, Jonathon, and Kyla.
- He is a friend and supporter.
- He is a thinker and believer.
- He is a rescuer, a survivor, and a risk taker.
- His nickname is "Cheeks"; he laughs easily and is cherished by many.

On August 28, 1998, Brian's bike fell from a trail, and his life changed in a heartbeat.

HOW DO WE KNOW WHAT THE TARGET IS?

The targeted outcome is a vision of the future shared by client and therapist and driven by the dream and desire of the individual. Dreams are unique to each individual, thus, targeted outcomes will also be. Therapists often ask: "Why targeted outcomes? Are we not being client-centered if we use short- and long-term goals?" A targeted outcome is the client's vision of the future related to occupational performance, yet not driven by time frames specific to the various clinical settings he or she may move through on route to its accomplishment. This is not to say that it is without a time frame. In fact, it becomes a dream with a deadline. Long-term goals are often thought of as the target. Short-term goals are the steps the therapist feels able to accomplish within the time frame that the client remains within a particular service. Therefore, short- and long-term goals become more therapist-driven than client-centered. The time frame for the targeted outcome is negotiated between client and therapist after consideration is given to the steps (action plans) required to achieve it. Targeted outcomes are directly related to the issues identified in the client's story, as narrated in Stage 1 of the OPPM. The outcome belongs to the individual and fits within the story of that client's life. Every occupation this individual now engages in on this journey has meaning to the client. We make paths rather than following paths already made. Thinking, feeling, and behaving this way puts occupation in context, which may indicate the need to completely revamp programs that do not reflect uniqueness and individuality in the populations for whom they were designed.

Defining the desired or targeted outcome addresses the questions "Where are we going?" and "How will we know when we get there?" Given the visionary process, we could ask clients to close their eyes and imagine how they would like life to be, paint the picture if you will. We, as therapists, can close our eyes, too, participate in the visualization, and use our knowledge, experience, task analysis expertise, and clinical reasoning to determine possibilities. We accept that clients and the networks that surround them also come with their brains, knowledge, problem-solving experience, imagination, and resilience. This is not something we get from a nominal or ordinal scale. Collaboration gives us the best of both client and therapist worlds. Clients need to have ownership in the plan. We make for more infallible plans when we use the expertise of all concerned. Negotiation refers to discussion, informed decision-making, exploration of options, and flexibility and agreement as to the time frames and content of the plan. Targeted outcomes are on a 1:1 ratio with the OPIs identified in Stage 1. For each OPI, there will be a targeted outcome. They are behaviorally stated and measurable, and they incorporate time frames considered to be reasonable by the individual.

TO WHOM DOES THE DREAM BELONG?

The dream belongs to the client, however, the therapist can play an active role in its development. Dreams are about an envisioned future, a future the client will live. Because the therapist will not live this future, he or she does not design it, but plays a part in the plan to attain it. Consider the client's dream as a garden. The individual chooses vegetables, herbs, flowers, shrubs, or some combination. Ideally, the therapist acts as a gardener, perhaps making recommendations for certain plants given the exposure. Together they cultivate the soil, dig the holes, plant, and water. The desired outcome is shared— the garden grows.

In a strong partnership, each member takes ownership and contributes in ways that do not duplicate but enhance each other. Thus, the therapist may act as a facilitator or potential catalyst.

> *[It is like the] meeting of two chemical substances:*
> *if there is any reaction, both are transformed.*
> (C.G. Jung)

DEVELOPING TARGETED OUTCOMES
AND ACTION PLANS

Brian: For me, the "dream with a deadline" consists of a picture of where I want to be. You have to fine-tune the picture as you go. I envision myself on a stage in front of a podium. I am wearing a denim shirt and denim shorts. My legs are skinny. I am speaking to an audience. (I can't see who it is or where it is yet.) I begin my speech to the audience by saying, "Four years ago, I had a spinal cord injury..." At this point, it is a process of refining the picture. Adding color, sound, mood, and feeling. You may have to adjust these elements, but this is my process of building the vision or dream.

In this case, the targeted outcome is to engage in public speaking within 4 years time. With the target in place, an action plan is developed that is a compilation of all possible modalities based in person (physical, cognitive, affective), occupation (adaptation or grading the related self-care, productivity, or leisure occupation), and environment (social, physical, cultural, and institutional) necessary to realize the goal (Canadian Association of Occupational Therapists [CAOT], 1997; Law, Cooper, Strong, Stewart, Rigby, & Letts, 1996). The theory we selected in Stage 2 that guided assessment and was confirmed in Stage 3, now directs intervention in Stage 5. So, for example, if we selected the biomechanical theory in Stage 2, we would expect to see biomechanical intervention in Stage 5.

Task analysis is the method used to design the step-by-step process involved in the development of the action plan. In determining the order of the items in the action plan, precedence is first given to skill building within "person." It would seem unfair to have an individual re-enter environments or occupations without strategies to resolve, minimize, or combat the personal components impeding his or her performance. If clients have made adaptations or developed skills in "person" previously, perhaps just a brief review in this area will be required. Once the plan for "person" is in place, consideration is given to "environmental" adaptation, support, or enhancement. "The client's environment contains aspects that are innocuous, threatening, accommodative, or supportive. Threatening or impeding aspects are changed while supportive elements are enhanced" (Matheson, 1998, p. 112). This is followed by graded entry or re-entry to the desired and meaningful "occupation." The Ecology of Human Performance Framework (Dunn, Brown, & McGuigan, 1994) supports this Person-Environment-Occupation (PEO) hierarchy and suggests five alternatives for therapeutic intervention:

1. **Establish or restore.** Remediate skills and abilities within "person"
2. **Alter.** Select "environments" that enable the person to perform with current skills and abilities
3. **Adapt.** Ongoing design of environments to fit performance in "occupation" (just right challenge)
4. **Prevent.** Predict lack of fit between PEO and intervene accordingly
5. **Create!**

Action plans are generated and negotiated by the client, associated clients, and therapist together in partnership. All parties may suggest possibilities within the categories of PEO. It is helpful if therapists explain intervention techniques in a way that clients can make informed decisions, while weaving in the clients' strengths and resources (Stage 4).

In Stage 5 of the OPPM, when collaborating on targeted outcomes and action plans, the questions of **what** and **who** need to be answered. Once the interventions related to person, environment, and occupation have been completed and agreed upon, we have answered the "what." We now go through the action plan a second time to determine "who" will carry out the various aspects of the plan. Additional players often provide the support, advocacy, and alliances needed to strengthen the likelihood of success. Matheson (1998) suggests taking this one step further. He proposes that once the goal list is made (in this case the targeted outcome and action plan), the client should make 20 copies and distribute them to family members, friends, colleagues, and treating professionals, as well as placing them in prominent locations. This is done as a means of demonstrating appreciation, commitment, and respect for targets generated. In all likelihood, it would also serve to engage and secure community involvement.

The time frames of targeted outcomes can often be negotiated up front, however, once the action plan has been set, consideration may once again be given to the realistic nature of the time frame necessary to complete it. Adjustment may be required. Time frames can also be assigned to the various steps of the action plan as a means of pacing and monitoring progress. An example of a targeted outcome and related action plan may be found in the case study in Chapter 10.

It is interesting to note that the components and conditions that may interfere with one occupation are in all likelihood to be the same barriers to performance in other occupations. Thus, by focusing on what has meaning to clients and developing action plans to resolve or overcome hurdles in one area, we may inadvertently work to improve occupational performance in other areas.

Doing Being Believing Becoming
(CAOT Promotional Campaign Slogan, 1999. Adapted from Wilcock, 1998.)

WHY IS BELIEVING IMPORTANT
AND HOW DOES IT RELATE TO STAGE 5?

One of the most obvious applications of believing lies in the arena of goal-setting and attainment. The future belongs to the client. Regardless of the length of time the therapist is involved in a rehabilitative relationship with the client and family, it remains only a snapshot of a bigger life in progress. Often, the term "negotiating" targets or outcomes with clients is used. Perhaps we should believe in the dreams and goals of clients and negotiate the means of attaining them.

BELIEVING BEGINS WITH HOPE

*Brian: They call me a C-5/ASIA/A, which refers to a classification of the level and type of spinal cord injury I sustained. It's interesting, even before I arrived in rehabilitation, it seemed that a picture had been painted about **what** I was. If they wanted preconceived ideas about me, it's too bad they weren't asking **who** I was. In that initial stage after the injury, I was devastated. I sank into a deep depression and had no sense of hope. Fear of the future completely overwhelmed me. I went to a dark place, and nothing was able to reach me there. Eventually, a turning point came, and I decided that I didn't want to be like this. I didn't want to accept and be what other people were telling me to be. I wanted to choose; I wanted to be in control of my life.*

Spencer, Davidson, and White (1997) describe hope as having cognitive, emotional, and spiritual elements. "The cognitive aspect of hope allows one to imagine possibilities and establish goals as well as to gauge limitations and test realities. Imagination and choice are crucial outgrowths of the cognitive aspects of hope" (p. 192). Rather than the daydreams and nightmares of imagination, clients hone wisely chosen challenges. The emotional aspects of hope are defined as having "distinction between basic or untested (unchallenged) hope and challenged hope. Unchallenged hope is analogous to wishful thinking that difficulties will magically disappear, whereas challenged hope acknowledges difficulties and develops positive beliefs and feelings about the future in which difficulties can be transcended" (p. 192). Hence, intention and will are outgrowths of the emotional aspects of hope (Spencer et al., 1997). Examinations of the spiritual nature of hope propose a conviction that one's life has purpose and meaning, either through one's inherent worth as an individual or connection to nature, other persons, or some larger entity (Spencer et al., 1997).

Brian: In my experience, the first step to developing hope was within the spiritual realm. With grief related to the past, a present I was unequipped to deal with, and a future that appeared foreboding, planning and setting goals was not yet appropriate. Perhaps one first needs to search for meaning. After much frightening reflection and suffering, a window opened that particular afternoon as determination that the future was going to be of my making was confirmed. I decided this is not who I am. I believe that anything is possible. I made a deal to try to think about a future of 1 year and stop focusing on death.

With an opening for hope in place, clients start to conceive possible futures. Imagination is now possible; the vision starts to develop ever so faintly. At this point, health care providers and all those who surround the client are pivotal in the promotion of choice and the power of believing in oneself. Whether hope begins in the cognitive, spiritual, or emotional realm probably will be different for each and every person and will be dependent on who they are as individuals. Whereas hope is tentative, possible, and yet insecure, belief is confident, strong, and sure. Thus, hope and belief do not necessarily travel hand-in-hand. Hope evolves into belief. We all probably prefer to be "believed in" rather than "hoped in."

> *Desire, Ask, Believe, Receive*
> (Stella Terrill Mann)

EMBRACING CHALLENGED HOPE

Individuals should be encouraged and dared to dream and not simply "make do" as a result of injury, illness, or disability. Imagine the devastating experience of having life take an abrupt turn as a result of injury or other health-related issues. Then add to this grief by being told directly or indirectly by health care practitioners that you can no longer be you. Previously held dreams, aspirations, and ambitions are now considered unrealistic and to hold on to these judged as living in denial. The meaning of denial is threefold, to assert that something is untrue, refusal to acknowledge, or refusal of a request (*Webster's Dictionary*, 1987). At times, we say that a client or family are "in denial," yet struggling to live with injury or illness every minute of every day. Given this relentless impact, we would be hard pressed to say they are refusing to acknowledge its existence. Perhaps they remain hopeful and encouraged by future prospects for a full life, a life of their design where beliefs and dreams matter.

Brian: Regardless of individual ability, a dream is a desired outcome or goal, something to shoot for. If you put your life on hold for that dream, you put yourself in a state of denial. For example, if I dream that I will walk one day, and I put my life on hold, waiting for that day to come, I am living in a state of denial. Dreaming can be just that—a dream. You can dream of success or wake up every day and be prepared to work hard for it. By developing plans and taking action in our lives, we can realize our dreams as an ongoing process, every day. Over time, dreams are realized, altered, changed, or, without action, they remain a wish. As you start to develop the vision, self-doubt lurks around the corner. Sometimes as confidence begins to build, the slightest bit of doubt projected by others in a tone of voice or facial expression can be enough to grab you by the toe and trip you up again, blocking that path to the future. When a baby is born, all the energy of the infant's family goes into nurturing the baby. In a healthy and loving environment, the family showers the child with positive affirmations and considers all the possibilities that lie ahead, rather than pondering all his or her possible shortcomings. Often, in a clinical setting, this falls to the wayside, and people are not treated as whole, but as a sum of individual parts, usually the parts that aren't working so well.

At times, clients are not believed in and struggle to find hope. Rather than support and unbiased and informed opportunities to make their own decisions, barriers may be presented by the very group that could be pivotal in the attainment of the dream. In Corring's and Cook's (1999) survey, clients discussed a sense of disillusionment with service providers. Particularly, they noted indifference to them as human beings, not being believed in, and lack of support. One individual sought "a pat on the back once in awhile instead of a kick in the back of the knees" (p. 76).

We have been taught to believe that negative equals realistic
and positive equals unrealistic.
(Susan Jeffers)

Many are concerned that this type of belief may be unrealistic or even detrimental to the well-being of clients and families as providing false hope. When we think about dreams, targets, or goals, they are future oriented and thus shrouded in mystery—something we can often only picture when we close our eyes. But if we can see it in this place, what possible harm is there in saying it out loud or asking help from others to attain it? As much can be gained from the process of the journey as from the final destination. As friend Pam Andrews, who carries the roles mother, partner, occupational therapy student, entrepreneur, and individual living with multiple sclerosis, once said, "Disability doesn't come with a handbook." Thus, we share tears of frustration; allow clients to change, modify, and determine the direction of the journey; and not only recognize but also celebrate successes along the way. Clients and therapists alike may have to learn to be patient yet undeterred. The outcome may, at times, be somewhat different than initially planned or not attained at all. But, if asked, all would likely agree.

You may be disappointed if you fail, but you are doomed if you don't try.
Being out on a limb is risky business, but that's where the fruit is.
(B. Sills)

Brian: When I was young, my father always said, "aim high." Needless to say, I was never a good pitcher. To me, this meant leave room for error, but take a chance at achieving a higher goal or outcome. Over the years, I have learned to focus on the target, keep my eyes on it, and keep working for it.

Encouragement is feedback.
(Kouzes and Posner)

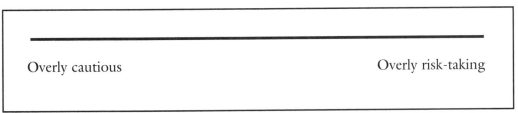

Figure 7-1. Continuum of risk taking.

MATCHES AND MISMATCHES

Believing in the dreams and destinies of clients involves some degree of risk-taking on the part of therapists. We all live our lives somewhat differently. What represents reasonable ambition to one may be anxiety-provoking for another. A challenge for one individual may be a threat to someone else. Remember that there is more than one way to cross the finish line, tortoises and hares can co-exist, both living successful, challenging, and stimulating lives. Rather than attempting to turn a client from the hare to the tortoise or from the tortoise to the hare, we are wise to recognize the person's inherent pace and adjust ours accordingly.

One of the barriers therapists put in the way of achieving client dreams is their own fear. Perhaps it is a fear of failure, a fear of reprisal, or maybe even a fear of success. One way to abate this fear is to remember the single word **competence**. If clients have not legally been deemed incompetent to make their own decisions, then they are competent and able to do so, even if it is not the decision therapists might make.

Take a moment to reflect. Are you a risk-taker or cautious by nature, or somewhere in between? Using an X, place yourself on the continuum (Figure 7-1), and consider the following questions: Would others place you in the same location on the continuum? What does it look like when an overly cautious therapist is linked to a risk-taking client? Or a risk-taking therapist paired with a cautious client?

This is about control. It is important to understand that these matches or mismatches are of our making. When we expect clients to change to match our comfort level, we hold control. With client dreams at stake, therapists must learn to trust both client and therapist capabilities and make the effort to match the client.

DOES BELIEVING REALLY MAKE A DIFFERENCE?

Imagine if belief in the dream was inherent in the partnership. Think of the empowerment. Imagine a team of people behind you, each bringing to the plan a different yet equally valuable component. First, the individual believes in self. This belief is shared by others. The therapist serves that belief by activating community resources and other interventions that will promote attainment of the target. With this type of group effort, it is difficult to visualize targets that could not be attained. "As professionals we must recognize their [clients'] tremendous vulnerability and offer them services in which they have choices and control" (Baum, 1980, p. 507). Occupational therapists have tremendous potential to believe and to develop the steps intended to move dreams to reality. This is what the targeted outcome and action plan of Stage 5 are all about.

> *Every blade of grass has its angel that bends over it and whispers "grow, grow."*
> **(The Talmud)**

WHAT DOES IT ALL MEAN?

We have talked at length in this chapter about the importance of believing in the dreams, targets, goals, and occupations of the client, as this is what gives meaning to life. When intervention is planned unilaterally by health care providers, it lacks meaning or fit, and individuals do not show up physically, mentally, emotionally, or spiritually. In essence, they vote with their feet. When therapists are bold enough to truly be with clients and whole-heartedly believe in their vision, mountains can be moved. Perhaps then,

(doing + being) x believing = becoming

"Our practice in the future should be evaluated not only on the basis of measurable, scientific outcomes, but also by what it contributes to the individual's human dignity, sense of mastery, and self-respect" (Yerxa, 1980).

With the vision and plan carefully laid out (being and believing), it now becomes a fluid process into the doing of Stage 6 and the eventual becoming (Stage 7) of the client.

ACKNOWLEDGMENTS

Jonathon Bell is Brian's 6-foot, 8-inch little brother and his acting hands at the moment. Thanks "Jody"!

REFERENCES

Baum, C. (1980). Occupational therapists put care in the health system. *American Journal of Occupational Therapy, 34*, 505-516.

Canadian Association of Occupational Therapists (1997). *Enabling occupation: An occupational therapy perspective.* Ottawa, Ontario, Canada: CAOT Publications ACE.

Corring, D., & Cook, J. (1999). Client-centred care means that I am a valued human being. *Canadian Journal of Occupational Therapy, 66*, 71-82.

Dunn, W., Brown, C., & McGuigan, A. (1994). The ecology of human performance: A framework for considering the effect of context. *American Journal of Occupational Therapy, 48*, 595-607.

Fearing, V.G., Law, M., & Clark, J. (1997). An occupational performance process model: Fostering client and therapist alliances. *Canadian Journal of Occupational Therapy, 64*, 7-15.

Law, M., Baptiste, S., Carswell, A., McColl, M.A., Polatajko, H., & Pollock, N. (1998). *The Canadian Occupational Performance Measure (COPM)* (3rd ed.). Ottawa, Ontario, Canada: CAOT Publications.

Law, M., Cooper, B., Strong, S., Stewart, D., Rigby, P., & Letts, L. (1996). The Person–Environment–Occupation model: A transactive approach to occupational performance. *Canadian Journal of Occupational Therapy, 63*, 9-23.

Matheson, L. (1998). Engaging the person in the process: Planning together for occupational therapy intervention. In M. Law (Ed.), *Client-Centered Occupational Therapy* (pp. 108-119). Thorofare, NJ: SLACK Incorporated.

Spencer, J., Davidson, H., & White, V. (1997). Helping clients develop hopes for the future. *American Journal of Occupational Therapy, 51*, 191-198.

Wilcock, A.A. (1998). Reflections on doing, being and becoming. *Canadian Journal of Occupational Therapy, 65*, 248-256.

Yerxa, E. (1980). Occupational therapy's role in creating a future climate of caring. *American Journal of Occupational Therapy, 34*, 529-534.

chapter eight

Stage 6

CONNECTING CLIENTS WITH THEIR FUTURE THROUGH OCCUPATION

JO CLARK, BSc(OT), OT(C)

> *Intervention is more than routinely implementing a list of tasks.*
> *Therapy turns into a story in a longer life story*
> *in which the therapist enters in the middle.*
> **(Mattingly, 1991)**

Previously, in Stage 5, the targeted outcome and the plan were developed. The targeted outcome tells us where we are going, and the action plan is a list of all possibilities in person, occupation, and environment (Law, Cooper, Strong, Stewart, Rigby, & Letts, 1996) that will move us toward that desired outcome. Once this list has been developed, negotiated, and confirmed by the client and therapist (the **what** of the plan), it is next determined **who** will carry out the various aspects of this plan.

In Stage 6, the plan is fine-tuned with definitions of the **when**, **where**, and **how** prior to initiating the implementation. **When** deals with questions related to timing and order. For example, do we start today or next week? What will we do first, and how long do we expect each aspect of the plan will take? Which modalities will follow second, third, and fourth? **Where** refers to the setting. Various aspects of the plan may be carried out in different environments, such as the client's home or community, work settings, or clinical settings. **How** concerns format, such as individual or group work, the degree of assistance needed, a procedural breakdown if you will. With this aspect of the plan now clearly defined, client and therapist alike can schedule the sessions needed to carry out joint responsibilities. Empowerment and commitment are rich with the clarity that this type of planning brings.

The Nike slogan "Just do it" is an apt description of the early part of Stage 6. The plan is finely tuned, refined, and then implemented with a variety of graded and meaningful steps in relation to person, environment, and occupation. Individuals who will be part of the plan have been identified and instructed as to the role they will play in this well-orchestrated construction. How, when, and where each portion of the intervention will be carried out has also been determined. This leaves little else to do but get started.

Most clients do so with a bang! Because everyone is so intimately involved in the negotiation and development of the plan, clients and families no longer remain passive in the process, with intervention imposed on them. Clients draft the design, and in combination with their expertise, that of occupational therapy and others, the plan is brought to life. This thorough and supportive process gives performance our best effort. Moving toward this "vision of the future anchors concrete problem-solving and therapeutic activities in a whole that is larger than the sum of its parts" (Spencer, Davidson, & White, 1997, p. 196).

INTERVENTION:
A MATTER OF CONTENT AND PROCESS

Although the idea of "just doing it" may be a way of thinking about engagement in intervention, the therapy itself is much more than this. Anyone can carry out a plan, but this is the testing ground of real life issues. Intervention is actually the clients' connection to their future, as it is in the doing that they are in touch with possibilities. Thus, much more than routine implementation, we carry out intervention with passion. Occupational therapists can role model believing and encouraging, while being sensitive to the reflection and reassessment clients may frequently experience. This period of therapy is an interchangeable combination of content and process. The content is what we do, the process is how we do it or how we feel about it. A client may work hard to practice and integrate energy conservation skills (content) while at the same time adapting to the notion of doing it in a different way (process). Recognition and validation of the feelings (embarrassment, frustration) that individuals may have about this change will be as valuable an aspect of the intervention as any of the content. Change needs to be accepted physically, mentally, and emotionally. Gender, culture, or age may give some clients the confidence to express these emotions freely. For others, the client-centered therapist will pick up on it in body language and give it the attention it deserves. The content of intervention needs to fit in the context of individual people and environments (cultural, social, and physical). Recommending bulky or complex equipment to a client who travels frequently, to a client who is cognitively unable to comprehend how to install and use it, or to a client who entertains frequently and is embarrassed by the presence of it, are examples of lack of congruency between content and process.

As clients begin to meet with success in the various steps of the action plan, confidence and acceptance build, while adaptation to new habits and patterns unfolds. Therapists will need to fine-tune the content/process equation throughout intervention while being diligent in their sensitivity to timing, fit, challenge, flow, and clients' self-perception and emotional well-being.

PROGRESS WILL BE INDIVIDUAL AND UNIQUE

Because individuals live in process, targets can shift, and progress may be variable rather than constant. Four possible progress scenarios are proposed for discussion in this chapter. In most cases, once the plan has been laid out, clients will start the intervention and progress at a consistent pace, ultimately achieving the targeted outcome. In certain circumstances, clients will meet with some degree of inertia at the onset of the intervention plan. However, with alteration and attention to process, these clients may begin and then progress in a pattern similar to the first group. Some clients may begin the process without incident and initially demonstrate progress. These individuals may meet stumbling blocks further along the route that will require a different type of fine-tuning to once again enable progress toward the desired outcome. Finally, some clients may decide through the course of intervention to discontinue and let go of the target. Figure 8-1 suggests possible problem-solving measures for a variety of routes to targeted outcomes.

As with any journey, change, new information, or unforeseen circumstances may cause us to reconsider and make alterations en route. Some of these alterations may slow us down or seemingly distract us from our destination as we attend to process. With a clear target ahead, we may forge into new or uncharted waters while wisely anticipating obstructions. At times, the voyage is smooth and unremarkable. At times, we may need to find different passageways. At times, the expedition is triumphant, and untouched lands are discovered. At times, regretfully, we may need to turn back. Whatever the outcome, the decision is always the client's. Remember a targeted outcome is never absolute, never a matter of pass or fail, rather a matter of clients' personal satisfaction.

SUCCESS IN MOST CASES

Flexibility, support, joy, and problem-solving are the key ingredients in the implementation phase. With a well-conceived plan, typically, individuals will actualize targeted outcomes with perhaps only slight alteration in time frames or modalities. Therapy can be painful, hard work, and at times very threatening for clients. It can also be filled with celebration, humor, and companionship, which may provide the leverage to progress and success. The wisdom we gain with experience tells us not only to applaud success related to content but also to the mastery of process. Success is attained if people are living in the moment and are happy to be where they are today. This enables people to be who they are in content and process. While it could be said that this may be an example of doing, being, and believing (Canadian Association of Occupational Therapists, 1999; Wilcock, 1998), we need to be mindful that becoming (the target) should not be at the expense of clients being who they are.

WHAT IF THE CLIENT IS NOT ABLE TO GET STARTED?

At times, by our very nature as occupational therapists, we are keen to "do" as we connect with clients. We are in this relationship by choice; clients, on the other hand, are often here by necessity. Hence, we must be sensitive to clients who are not yet ready to take action. Often when dealing with illness, injury, loss, or change, clients must have an

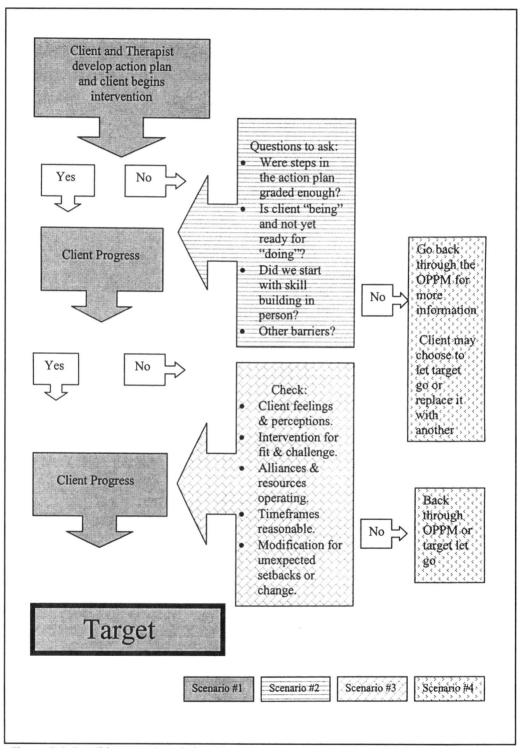

Figure 8-1. Possible scenarios of client progress.

opportunity to "be" before coming to terms with their future. Spencer, Davidson, and White (1997) emphasize the importance of honoring this process and recognizing that acknowledging grief and despair is often much more important than pushing clients toward goals prematurely. This process of reflection that each client experiences is only constant in one way—it will be inconsistent from individual to individual in both duration and presentation. Cognitively and physically, we may work toward a certain goal, while emotionally and spiritually the essence or soul of the individual client quietly encourages to simply follow what feels right. Labeling this as lack of motivation or non-compliance is a missed opportunity to be in process with clients. Some individuals do not come from a goal-oriented background, and, therefore, they may not have the instinct to be focused on the future.

When inertia is experienced at the onset, it is prudent to investigate with the client whether the steps are graded finely enough to allow for immediate success. Perhaps the individual feels overwhelmed with fear of failure while facing this first milestone. Conversely, fear of success and a future that remains foreign may be the barrier. Either way, it is of utmost importance to connect with clients, draw upon their strengths and resources, and support them through this process. Inertia can also be experienced when skill building in the person has been overlooked as a first step. When individuals return to previous environments and occupations without new skills, performance issues are resurrected. Additional questions can be asked related to timing issues, other barriers, or variables overlooked in the development of the plan. These can be addressed and woven into the plan at this time. As with every other aspect of the Occupational Performance Process Model, it is important that therapists do not try to troubleshoot in the absence of the client. It is too easy to ignore or make judgments and assumptions about the origin of the inaction. Troubleshooting in partnership and once again allowing the client to direct the process proves beneficial.

VARIATIONS IN PROGRESS AND POSSIBLE NEED FOR MODIFICATION

Sometimes during the enactment of the steps toward the targeted outcome, clients recognize that the original vision, or means of getting there, may need alteration. Unexpected obstacles may present themselves, or resources may become depleted. Other changes in person-environment-occupation variables may cause a temporary or long-term change of focus or result in reconsideration of the plan. It is at these moments that individuals need the greatest degree of support, encouragement, and validation. Whether to simply pause, reflect, and eventually continue on the same occupational path in a graded or adapted fashion or to discontinue the journey is ultimately the choice of the client. Hopefully, therapists' first inclination is to become creative barrier busters, clearing debris from the path, reassuring the traveler, and motivating success. Appropriate use of humor can be an effective way to empower clients and create balance and perhaps needed levity. Taking a reading of client's perceptions and feelings will also provide pertinent information. You may find that these perceptions are not based on factual information from all perspectives. Perhaps the individual is fatigued and simply needs to pause and rest. Perhaps self-perceptions are filled more with "can't do" than "can do." Listening provides opportunity not only for ventilation but validation. Successes already accomplished can be reaffirmed and support provided.

It may be necessary to review the grading of the steps in the plan. When progress becomes difficult to witness or monitor in the midst of intervention, it may be that the gaps between the steps are too wide. Matheson (1998) states that "roles that are overwhelming can lead to decompensation, erosion of self-efficacy with attendant decrease in risk-taking behavior, exploration, and curiosity" (p. 113). Failure can at times be a healthy part of the rehabilitation process. As long as failure is incorporated as a learning experience and identified as a consequence of remediable factors, decompensation and erosion of self-efficacy will be limited (Matheson, 1998). Replacement of depleting resources, alteration to time frames, or other modifications may also be required at this point.

CHANGE OF PLAN...TARGET LET GO

Although clients may struggle and be pushed outside of their comfort zone on the intervention path, it is always important to allow them to own the process. Whether they choose to pursue or discontinue is up to them and may be based in their comfort with risk-taking behavior. The last thing needed at this point is advice. When frustration sets in, it may be wise to encourage individuals to take a break and avoid impulsive decisions. If the client decides to let the vision go or to replace it with another, it is time to adjourn from the "doing" and "be" with the individual. These are huge life decisions in many cases and are not to be glossed over lightly. Clients will need time to grieve. Rushing in to replace the target with another and return to "doing" may be a mistake. Taking the time to support the emotional process for another may be the most therapeutic intervention in which we engage. Implementation in partnership means we not only encourage each other along the way, but also celebrate successes and share a natural process of grieving related to accepting loss.

BENEFITS OF INTERVENTION DIRECTED TOWARD TARGETED OUTCOMES AND BASED ON ACTION PLANS

Therapists who develop plans that do not have meaning to clients, or refine steps to the extent that clients cannot determine the purpose of certain activities (stacking cones), bear responsibility for convincing clients regarding the need for occupational therapy. With the development of targeted outcomes and action plans, which are well organized and based in desired activity, ownership in implementation shifts to the client. Individuals often become so motivated that targets are met before expected or surpassed altogether. Rebeiro and Miller Polgar (1999) suggest that client-driven selection of meaningful occupation and therapist enablement of the just right challenge (demands of occupation = skills of individual) influence optimal experience, flow, occupational performance, and life satisfaction for those with disability. The author has experienced a situation whereby, after the development of the action plan with the client and definition as to how it would be carried out, the client hugged this therapist and asked for a copy of the plan. With initiative, responsibility, and confidence shifted to the client, this individual was routinely waiting at the door, eager to get started. Not only did she meet her goal, she also surpassed it within a week. No one, including the client herself, could believe the difference. As Spencer, Davidson, and White (1997) state: "One of our unique capabilities as occupational therapists is the provision of opportunities for meaningful doing that can become transforming experiences, thereby creating a belief in possibilities that were thought lost or were never imagined" (p. 197). If the client is an organization, the same principles apply. Let the members own possibilities, thereby facilitating a process of helping groups to help themselves. These skills make occupational therapists well-placed as leaders in problem-solving facilitation.

COMMUNICATING INTERVENTION AND TIME FRAMES TO THE TEAM

Because approximate time frames can be estimated for each of the steps of the action plan, it is particularly helpful with respect to planning among clients and teams. It doesn't matter if the client is an adult or a child, a group or an organization. Clarifying intervention strategies, time frames, responsible parties, and the required settings will prove to enhance team coordination and communication toward outcomes directed by clients. When clients are treated as truly unique beings, services are tailored to fit their individual and collective needs. If there is not a fit between what the individual needs and what is offered, rather than reshaping people, we reshape and revamp the services meant to support them. For the most part, the fulfillment of the plan will be a fluid process, and individualized client interventions will fit in the continuum of services offered. For example, clients may move from one setting to another partway through intervention. When the plan is well-organized and clearly articulated, continuity and seamless transition for clients is achieved.

"JUST DOCUMENT IT"—PROGRESS NOTES

Client-centered practice is reflected in documentation that is free of labels, judgment, and generalities or unrelated information. Once the targeted outcome has been set and the action plan determined, monitoring and recording progress is made easy. Progress notes reflect what has been completed and what is yet to be done. Note progress related to the expected time frames. Note any incidental information that is pertinent to changes in the plan or the target. You are now able to freely share the content of progress notes and reports with clients and caregivers. You are documenting their dreams and their hopes; this will not be a surprise to them. Given the extremely collaborative and equitable nature of the process, it would not be unreasonable to visualize clients recording their own progress.

CONCLUSION

Once this type of recipe has been developed, the beauty is that anyone can carry out the plan. Should therapists be absent and replaced during portions of intervention or clients transition to new settings, continuity is made easy. Remembering that there may be a number of ways to reach the same end with variations to either content or process, intervention is viewed as more than simply carrying out a predetermined set of steps. It is not only what the client is doing, but also the meaning of that doing, that has relevance. Taking action on the plan links clients to their future and becomes not only the route to the future but the testing ground where dreams may or may not become realities. Therapists need to be prepared to engage in both ends of the spectrum—celebration of achievement and support of grief related to setbacks—and to do so with passion. The journey of rehabilitation can at times be an adventure, unpredictable yet rewarding. Acknowledgment and validation of the pain associated with potential loss of occupation and meaning is critical to client-centered occupational therapy practice. Simply resolving functional issues is secondary in importance to the emotional process of helping individuals to regroup and imagine new futures when original targets are not attained. When clients are emotionally ready to consider new targets, the process can be initiated once again. At the completion of Stage 6, clients move on to Stage 7 where outcomes are measured. An example of intervention implementation and documentation can be found in Chapter 10.

REFERENCES

Canadian Association of Occupational Therapists (CAOT). (1999). Promotional campaign slogan. (See Wilcock, 1998.)

Law, M., Cooper, B., Strong, S., Stewart, D., Rigby, P., & Letts, L. (1996). The Person–Environment–Occupation model: A transactive approach to occupational performance. *Canadian Journal of Occupational Therapy, 63*, 9-23.

Matheson, L. (1998). Engaging the person in the process: Planning together for occupational therapy intervention. In M. Law (Ed.), *Client-Centered Occupational Therapy* (pp. 108-119). Thorofare, NJ: SLACK Incorporated.

Mattingly, C. (1991). The narrative nature of clinical reasoning. *American Journal of Occupational Therapy, 45*, 998-1005.

Rebeiro, K., & Miller Polgar, J. (1999). Enabling occupational performance: Optimal experiences in therapy. *Canadian Journal of Occupational Therapy, 66*, 14-22.

Spencer, J., Davidson, H., & White, V. (1997). Helping clients develop hopes for the future. *American Journal of Occupational Therapy, 51*, 191-198.

Wilcock, A.A. (1998). Reflections on doing, being and becoming. *Canadian Journal of Occupational Therapy, 65*, 248-256.

chapter nine

EVALUATING CLIENT PERFORMANCE RELATED TO TARGETED OUTCOMES

MARY EGAN, PHD, OT(C), CLAIRE-JEHANNE DUBOULOZ, PHD, OT(C)

A 5-year-old boy with coordination problems plays his first game of catch with his dad. A recently widowed octogenarian organizes meal preparation and house cleaning. An accountant battling depression plans strategies to manage her work. Every day, occupational therapists help clients identify and work toward goals related to meaningful activities in their daily lives.

The Occupational Performance Process Model (OPPM) (Fearing, Law, & Clark, 1997) is used to assist clients to achieve their occupational goals. The process begins with Stage 1, in which the client and therapist identify occupational performance issues (OPIs). A theoretical approach is selected in Stage 2. In Stage 3, components and environmental conditions contributing to the OPIs are identified. The strengths and resources available to the client and therapist are identified in Stage 4. The client's vision of the future, in terms of occupation, is articulated in behavioral terms in Stage 5, and a time line for the attainment of this vision is negotiated. The plan is implemented through occupation in Stage 6. Finally, in Stage 7, the therapist and client determine whether or not the desired results have been obtained.

Measurement of the attainment of targeted occupational outcomes provides valuable feedback and may assist the client and therapist to identify further goal areas (Fearing et al., 1997). Evaluation of targeted outcomes can also be extremely helpful in justifying occupational therapy service delivery in today's competitive health care system (de Clive-Lowe, 1996). However, methods used must allow occupational therapists to report the level of achievement of targeted outcomes at both the patient and program level. As well, results must be interpretable by other members of the treatment team, administration, and third party payers.

Evaluation of targeted outcomes can be somewhat intimidating at first. What tools should be used? How often should evaluation take place? These are among the many questions facing occupational therapists preparing to evaluate and report the outcomes of intervention. The goals of this chapter are to briefly define outcome evaluation and to outline methods that can be used to evaluate the attainment of client-specific targeted outcomes at both the client and program level.

EVALUATION OF OUTCOME—
WHAT IT IS AND WHAT IT ISN'T

Watching the achievements of our clients each day, it is difficult to believe that any-one could imagine that our interventions are not effective. Such confidence in the out-come of services provided is not unique to occupational therapy. In fact, health care pro-fessionals are often so sure that what they do works that their evaluations of practice often focus on content (who and what is used to provide the service), process (how service is provided), and output (how many units of service are provided), rather than the outcome of intervention. Outcome refers to the results of service for the client (Wood-Dauphinee, Arsenault, & Richards, 1994).

Outcome is generally more difficult to evaluate than content, process, or output. Rather than just describing what is done during intervention, the therapist must look for evidence of a change in the client as a result of service. This requires that the client be assessed prior to and following intervention. But how should this assessment be carried out?

Occupational therapists often summarize their work as the enhancement of function (Turner, 1996). Measurement of independence in basic daily functioning before and after intervention has therefore been recommended as an important component of occupa-tional therapy intervention specifically, and rehabilitation in general (Ware, Phillips, Yody, & Adamczyk, 1996). Several measures of daily functioning, such as the Functional Inde-pendence Measures (FIM) (Keith, Granger, Hamilton, & Sherwin, 1987), have been developed and adopted into standard patient assessment and reassessment protocols. Such measures of general function are well-recognized by other members of the treat-ment team and seem to cover a wide variety of patient goals. Some are used routinely so that institutions can report on average patient outcomes (Hamilton, Granger, Sherwin, Zielezny, & Tashman, 1987).

However, occupational therapists know that clients and their goals are so different from one another that a "one size fits all" approach to outcome evaluation does not capture the true results of intervention. Occupational therapists practicing from a client-centered per-spective are also aware that not all clients share the same definition of enhanced function (Carson, 1999). For instance, a positive outcome for one client might entail organizing help with bathing, dressing, and personal hygiene to conserve energy so that he can carry on with his work. Such an individual would be considered dependent in activities of daily liv-ing. His score on a traditional measure of function such as the FIM would be relatively low, indicating a poor outcome. From the client's perspective, this would be simply not true.

But how can the client's unique goals be considered when measuring outcomes? Wouldn't the therapist require an encyclopedic knowledge of self-care, productivity, and leisure evaluations? And if different assessments are used, how can client outcomes be compiled to allow reporting of the general effectiveness of occupational therapy pro-grams? Only a generic outcome evaluation of occupational performance would meet these two criteria. Fortunately, such evaluations do exist. Two of the most widely used and highly regarded, the Canadian Occupational Performance Measure (COPM) and Goal Attainment Scaling (GAS), will be described.

CLIENT-CENTERED MEASURES OF OCCUPATIONAL PERFORMANCE

COPM

The COPM (Law, Baptiste, Carswell, McColl, Polatajko, & Pollock, 1998) was developed as a non-diagnosis-specific method of evaluating change in occupational performance from a client-centered perspective. This tool guides the client and therapist through a process of identifying OPIs and evaluating their performance and their satisfaction with this performance both before and after occupational therapy intervention.

As outlined in Chapter 3, four steps are involved when using the COPM (Law et al., 1998). First, OPIs are identified. The occupational therapist interviews the client regarding the occupations he or she wants to do, must do, or is expected to do over the course of a day. Second, the client is prompted to rate the importance of each of the occupations on a scale from 1 (not important at all) to 10 (extremely important). Third, the client is asked to reflect on these ratings and identify up to five occupational issues on which he or she would like to focus. Once this is done, the client is asked to rate both his or her present performance and satisfaction with this performance on a scale from 1 to 10. At a time then agreed upon by the occupational therapist and client, performance and satisfaction are reassessed. Comparison of this post-therapy score with the pre-therapy scores allows the therapist and client to quantify changes that occurred over the course of therapy.

For example, Jane, a 35-year-old computer professional, became an occupational therapy client during an in-patient rehabilitation stay for acute rheumatoid arthritis. With her occupational therapist, Paul, she completed the COPM prior to the start of intervention. Jane identified two priority areas:

1. Computer access (Jane developed disabling pain in her wrist after 30 minutes of using a regular mouse)
2. Caring for her dogs (Jane and her husband raise Labrador retrievers and have 12 dogs in their kennel)

Jane rated her level of performance and satisfaction in these areas before and immediately following 2 weeks of intensive occupational therapy during which she and Paul experimented with different computer access tools and energy conservation methods related to caring for the dogs. To determine the amount of change in performance, Paul added the pre-intervention performance scores and divided by the number of OPIs. The same was done to determine the change in satisfaction. The total for all performance scores following intervention was summed and divided by the number of OPIs. The same was done for post-intervention satisfaction scores. Comparison of scores before and after occupational therapy indicated an increase in both performance and satisfaction following intervention (Table 9-1).

To ensure accurate and useful measurement of change, the evaluation tool utilized must be reliable, valid, sensitive to clinically important amounts of change, and easy to use. Reliability refers to the stability of the score over various testing conditions. That is,

Table 9-1
Results of COPM Pre- and Post-Intervention—Jane

OPIs
1. Accessing computer

Importance	Time 1 (Pre-Intervention)		Time 2 (Post-Intervention)	
	Performance	Satisfaction	Performance	Satisfaction
10	2	2	8	7

2. Caring for dogs

Importance	Time 1 (Pre-Intervention)		Time 2 (Post-Intervention)	
	Performance	Satisfaction	Performance	Satisfaction
10	3	3	5	7

Performance 1 = 5/2 = 2.5   Satisfaction 1 = 5/2 = 2.5
Performance 2 = 13/2 = 6.5   Satisfaction 2 = 14/2 = 7

if no real change has occurred, does the tool give the same result each time it is used (i.e., test-retest reliability) and when different individuals administer the test (interrater reliability)? Good test-retest reliability has been demonstrated (Law & Stewart, 1996; Sanford, Law, Swanson, & Guyatt, 1994), however, no reports of interrater reliability are available.

Validity refers to the degree to which the tool measures the concept it is intended to measure. Both criterion (the extent to which scores obtained using the tool are similar to scores from tools traditionally used to measure the same concept) and construct validity (the extent to which one finds theoretical support for measures from the tool) have been demonstrated by the authors and others (e.g., Bosch, 1995). Responsiveness to change has also been documented (Law, Polatajko, Pollock, McColl, Carswell, & Baptiste, 1994; Mirkopoulos & Butler, 1994; Wilcox, 1994).

The authors report that the COPM has been used successfully with clients as young as 7 years old (Law et al., 1998). In situations where a client has difficulty responding to the questions, it is recommended that the therapist attempt to obtain what input he or she can and then to confer with individuals who may also be involved in the intervention (e.g. parents, teachers, caregivers) (Law et al., 1998).

GAS

The GAS is another method of measuring change in client-specific goals. Originally developed to measure change resulting from participation in mental health treatment programs (Kiresuck & Sherman, 1968), the GAS has since been used by a wide variety of health professionals to evaluate diverse health outcomes. Essentially, the process allows the therapist and the client to identify therapy goals, rate the desirability of potential outcomes, and compare performance in these goal areas pre- and post-intervention.

$$\text{GAS} = 50 + 10 \times \frac{\Sigma(\text{weight of each goal} \times \text{attainment score for that goal})}{\sqrt{[.7 \times \Sigma(\text{weight of each goal})^2 + .3(\Sigma\text{weights of each goal})^2]}}$$

Figure 9-1. GAS formula.

Six steps are used to identify the GAS score (Stolee, Rockwood, Fox, & Streiner, 1992). First, the areas of functioning that will be goal areas for the client are identified. Second, a weight reflecting the importance of each of the goal areas is assigned. Typically, weights of 1 (least important) to 9 (most important) are used. Third, the expected time to goal attainment is determined, using professional judgment and the client's expectations. Fourth, a typical successful outcome of intervention is identified and given a score of 0. Fifth, other potential outcomes are identified and scored according to whether they reflect an outcome much worse than expected (-2), somewhat worse than expected (-1), somewhat better than expected (1), or much better than expected (2). Using the formula in Figure 9-1, the GAS score is then determined. The formula is used to provide a standardized score, with 50 corresponding to average goal attainment when the GAS is used with a relatively large number of clients. With a relatively large number of clients, the standard deviation among client GAS scores would be 10.

Scoring is carried out both at the initiation and the completion of intervention. The change score is reported as the post-intervention GAS score minus the pre-intervention GAS score.

Traditionally, GAS has been used to measure progress on any type of treatment goal. That is, goals have not been exclusively occupational in nature. As well, identification of goal areas and weighting and scoring of goals has been done by the treatment team without input of the client (Rockwood, Joyce, & Stolee, 1997). To ensure that GAS is used in an occupation-focused, client-centered manner, the therapist must remember to ensure that goals relate to occupational performance areas (e.g., productivity, self-care, leisure activities) rather than performance components (e.g., memory, strength). As well, therapists must ensure that clients are active in goal identification, weighting, and scoring.

The following is an example of the use of GAS to evaluate targeted outcomes. Glen, a 72-year-old retired bank manager, began seeing an occupational therapist on the recommendation of his family physician. He had previously been active in many activities including golfing, delivering meals on wheels, and studying the history of early Canada. However, following the death of his wife, Glen found himself having difficulty just getting up in the morning. He had experienced significant weight loss, due, in part he felt, to the fact that he was not motivated to shop, cook, or go out for meals. With his occupational therapist, Noor, Glen identified and rated the importance of the following OPIs:

- Meal preparation (importance rating = 9)
- Reading (importance rating = 5)

$$\text{GAS pre-} = \frac{50 + 10 \times [(9 \text{x-}1) + (5 \text{x-}2)]}{\sqrt{[.7 \times (9^2 + 5^2) + .3(9 + 5)^2]}} = 33.5$$

$$\text{GAS post-} = \frac{50 + 10 \times [(9 \text{x}1) + (5 \text{x}0)]}{\sqrt{\equiv[.7 \times (9^2 + 5^2) + .3(9 + 5)^2]}} = 57.8$$

Change score = 57.8 - 33.5 = 24.3

Figure 9-2. GAS pre- and post-intervention—Glen.

Noor and Glen determined that significant progress should be made in these areas within 3 weeks of twice-weekly therapy sessions. Glen wished to concentrate on preparing lunch, as he felt best around the noon hour. Noor and Glen then determined that the outcome of these sessions would be considered successful if Glen was preparing lunch at least 4 days a week (score of 0). A somewhat more successful outcome would be preparation of lunch 5 to 6 days a week (score of 1). A much more successful outcome would be preparation of lunch 7 days a week (score of 2). Unsuccessful outcomes included preparation of lunch 1 to 3 days a week (score of -1) and preparation of lunch 0 days (score of -2).

Glen had formerly enjoyed reading in the evenings. Noor and Glen decided that a successful outcome would consist of reading 3 nights a week (score of 0). Other outcomes were scored in a manner similar to that above (i.e., 0 nights [score of -2], 1 to 2 nights [score of -1], 4 to 5 nights [score of 1], 6 to 7 nights [score of 2]).

During the week prior to the start of intervention, Glen had made lunch once and had not read at all. During the week following intervention, Glen prepared lunch five times and read 3 nights. Calculation and comparison of GAS scores pre- and post-interventions are outlined in Figure 9-2. The post-intervention GAS represents a slightly better than average outcome. Comparison of the pre- and post-intervention GAS scores demonstrates a positive change in Glen's occupational performance.

To date, psychometric testing of the GAS, with goal identification and scoring done primarily by health care professionals, has been performed. Under these conditions, there is evidence of good interrater reliability of GAS scores of physicians and nurses (Stolee et al., 1992). When used to assess progress in individuals receiving inpatient rehabilitation for central nervous system disorders, including traumatic brain injury and stroke, and individuals treated on specialized geriatric units, moderate to good correlation was obtained between change scores observed using accepted measures of ADL and IADL functioning and GAS. As well, GAS provided greater responsiveness to change than these measures (Rockwood et al., 1997; Rockwood, Stolee, & Fox, 1993). While it is likely that good reliability, validity, and responsiveness to change would also be noted with GAS used in a more client-centered fashion, this has yet to be determined.

At the present time, the GAS is perhaps better recognized by other health professionals than the COPM. However, there are at least four potential disadvantages to this method compared with the COPM. First, as stated previously, professionals using GAS have traditionally developed goal areas and ratings independent of the client (Rockwood et al., 1997). Therefore, while the GAS has allowed the identification of a general score reflecting unique client needs, it has not been client-directed. Team members who have used the GAS with this conventional method may have difficulty implementing such a change.

Second, the traditional GAS format is structured to allow goal-setting in any area. That is, it lacks prompts to remind the occupational therapist and client to focus on occupational performance areas of productivity, self-care, and leisure. Without such reminders, the client and therapist may stray into performance component issues, such as physical and mental functioning.

Third, gradations of success must be identified during the initial assessment. This process can be quite time-consuming. Finally, scoring of the GAS uses a more complicated mathematical formula. The scores themselves are therefore more difficult to calculate and to explain than the more straightforward COPM scores.

LESS FORMAL METHODS OF EVALUATING TARGETED OUTCOMES

We strongly recommend that targeted outcomes be evaluated using one of the methods described above. However, we realize that use of a formal tool can be intimidating at first. Outcomes could be evaluated using a less formal method consisting of the following steps:

1. During the initial stages of intervention, ask the client to identify his or her major OPIs (e.g., by asking a question such as, "What are the activities that you most want to work on figuring out ways to accomplish?"). Then, with the client, define targeted outcomes related to these issues. For example, an individual experiencing hip and neck pain due to osteoarthritis identifies difficulty attending practices of a community choir as his major OPI. The targeted outcome of occupational therapy is that he will be able to participate in the weekly 3-hour practice by the end of 2 weeks.

2. Review the targeted outcomes with the client at a predetermined reassessment time. Ask the client if these goals have been achieved.

This kind of general questioning is a less structured form of outcome evaluation than use of tools such as the COPM. Degrees of goal attainment will not be apparent, and it will be difficult for you to compare attainment of targeted outcomes among your clients.

However, you will obtain a better indication of your clients' goals and achievements than if you had not asked these questions. For many therapists, this step provides a first stop on the way to using tools such as the COPM in their daily practice.

DEMONSTRATING THAT OCCUPATIONAL THERAPY MAKES A DIFFERENCE

After just a month of using the COPM, you are very positive about the results. Many clients have demonstrated remarkable changes in their performance and satisfaction with this performance over the course of intervention. In situations where clients did not rate themselves as having changed, use of the COPM helped form the basis of important discussions about short- and long-term goals, different ways of being "independent," dealing with loss, and reconstructing hope. In fact, after reviewing pre- and post-intervention results for 25 clients, you are ready to go to the media with the exciting news that occupational therapy definitely leads to positive changes in daily occupations.

But do score increases on the COPM before and after intervention allow a therapist to state unequivocally that occupational therapy produced the changes documented? The answer to this question is a qualified no. A positive difference in the COPM scores (or scores from any other evaluation) following intervention just demonstrates that the client changed during this time. This change may have been the result of maturation, spontaneous recovery, other interventions received at the same time, or anything else that happened between the beginning and end of occupational therapy intervention. Strong evidence that occupational therapy made the difference can only be obtained by ruling out these possibilities through, for example, use of a control group of similar clients who did not participate in occupational therapy.

It should also be remembered that even when change in occupational performance has occurred, it may not be maintained or carried over into a new environment. The latter may be particularly problematic if therapy has taken place in an institutional environment prior to the client returning home (Egan, Warren, Hessel, & Gilewich, 1992). To ensure that intervention has resulted in lasting change, further reassessment must be carried out at a later date in the client's environment.

However, while pre- and post-intervention assessment of targeted outcomes does not unequivocally prove the effectiveness of occupational therapy, it does furnish the therapist with convincing evidence of the value of intervention to administrators and third party payers. As well, it ensures that client-centered outcomes drive the therapeutic process. By using client-centered measures to evaluate and report the outcome of intervention goals, both client and therapist can celebrate their success attaining unique and valued goals.

REFERENCES

Bosch, J. (1995). *The reliability and validity of the Canadian Occupational Performance Measure*. Unpublished master's thesis. McMaster University, Hamilton, Ontario, Canada.

Carson, R. (1999). Client-centred practice in an American acute care rehabilitation hospital: A case study. *Occupational Therapy Now, 1*(3), 5-7.

de Clive-Lowe, S. (1996). Outcome measurement, cost-effectiveness and clinical audit: The importance of standardised assessment to occupational therapists in meeting these new demands. *British Journal of Occupational Therapy, 59*, 357-362.

Egan, M., Warren, S.A., Hessel, P.A., & Gilewich, G. (1992). Activities of daily living following hip fracture. *Occupational Therapy Journal of Research, 12*, 342-356.

Fearing, V.G., Law, M., & Clark, J. (1997). An occupational performance process model: Fostering client and therapist alliances. *Canadian Journal of Occupational Therapy, 64*, 7-15.

Hamilton, B.B., Granger, C.V., Sherwin, F.S., Zielezny, M., & Tashman, J.S. (1987). A uniform national data system for medical rehabilitation. In M.J. Fuhrer (Ed.), *Rehabilitation Outcomes: Analysis and Measurement* (pp. 137-147). Baltimore: Paul H. Brookes.

Keith, R.A., Granger, C.V., Hamilton, B.B., & Sherwin, F.S. (1987). The Functional Independence Measure: A new tool for rehabilitation. In M.G. Eisenberg & R.C. Grzesiak (Eds.), *Advances in Clinical Rehabilitation* (Vol. 1, pp. 6-18). New York: Springer-Verlag.

Kiresuck, T.J., & Sherman, R.E. (1968). Goal attainment scaling: A general method for evaluating comprehensive community mental health programs. *Community Mental Health Journal, 4*, 443-453.

Law, M., Baptiste, S., Carswell, A., McColl, M.A., Polatajko, H., & Pollock, N. (1998). *Canadian Occupational Performance Measure (COPM)* (3rd ed.) Ottawa, Ontario, Canada: CAOT Publications.

Law, M., Polatajko, H., Pollock, N., McColl, M.A., Carswell, A., & Baptiste, S. (1994). The Canadian Occupational Performance Measure: Results of pilot testing. *Canadian Journal of Occupational Therapy, 61*, 191-197.

Law, M., & Stewart, D. (1996). *Test retest reliability of the COPM with children*. Unpublished manuscript. McMaster University School of Rehabilitation Science, Hamilton, Ontario, Canada.

Mirkopoulos, C., & Butler, K. (1994). *Quality assurance: Clients' perceptions of goal performance and satisfaction*. Proceedings of the 11th World Congress of Occupational Therapy. London, England.

Rockwood, K., Joyce, B., & Stolee, P. (1997). Use of Goal Attainment Scaling in measuring clinically important change in cognitive rehabilitation patients. *Journal of Clinical Epidemiology, 50*, 581-588.

Rockwood, K., Stolee, P., & Fox, R.A. (1993). Use of Goal Attainment Scaling in measuring clinically important change in the frail elderly. *Journal of Clinical Epidemiology, 46*, 1113-1118.

Sanford, J., Law, M., Swanson, L., & Guyatt, G. (1994). *Assessing clinically important change as an outcome of rehabilitation in older adults*. Paper presented at the Conference of the American Society of Aging, San Francisco.

Stolee, P., Rockwood, K., Fox, R.A., & Streiner, D.L. (1992). The use of Goal Attainment Scaling in a geriatric care setting. *Journal of the American Geriatrics Society, 40*, 574-578.

Turner, A. (1996). The philosophy and history of occupational therapy. In A.Turner, M. Foster, & S.E. Johnson (Eds.), *Occupational Therapy and Physical Dysfunction* (4th ed., pp. 3-25). London: Churchill Livingstone.

Ware, J.E., Phillips, J., Yody, B.B., & Adamczyk, J. (1996). Assessment tools: Functional health status and patient satisfaction. *American Journal of Medical Quality, 11*, S50-S53.

Wilcox, A. (1994). *A study of verbal guidance for children with developmental coordination disorder*. Unpublished master's thesis. University of Western Ontario, London, Ontario.

Wood-Dauphinee, S., Arsenault, A.B., & Richards, C.L. (1994). Outcome assessment in rehabilitation. Overview of the 2nd National Rehabilitation Conference. *Canadian Journal of Rehabilitation, 7*, 171-184.

chapter ten

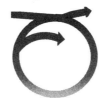

Case Study: A Demonstration of the Occupational Performance Process Model

Jo Clark, BSc(OT), OT(C)

The preceding chapters of Section II outlined the methods and beliefs of the seven stages of the Occupational Performance Process Model (OPPM) (Fearing, Law, & Clark, 1997). This chapter will apply the OPPM through a case study. This portion of the book may be used to guide applications in practice and provide possibilities in documentation. As previously stated, the OPPM provides a guideline, a process to think about the provision of client-centered occupational therapy services. It is not a prescription. Although this process model may be applied to practice with all types of clients (children, families, adults, groups, organizations), for the purpose of this example, we will revisit our client, Lisa, whom we first met in Chapter 4. The reader is encouraged to refer to previous chapters for more information on each of the stages as Lisa and her occupational therapist work through the process together.

CASE STUDY: LISA

Lisa is a 27-year-old woman who has experienced a depressive reaction following the birth of her second child. She returned home after the birth of the new baby, and within 2 weeks, she was readmitted to mental health services. At that time, she was uncommunicative, emotional, and withdrawn. Her mother has come to stay and is looking after the new baby and the 2-year-old while Lisa is in the hospital. Lisa has 6 months of maternity leave before returning to her job as a legal secretary. Her discharge is planned for the end of the week, and everyone is wondering how Lisa will manage at home. In particular, there is concern about how Lisa will fulfill the occupational requirements of caring for her children. An occupational therapy assessment has been requested.

STAGE 1—NAME, VALIDATE, PRIORITIZE OCCUPATIONAL PERFORMANCE ISSUES

The Canadian Occupational Performance Measure (COPM) (Law, Baptiste, Carswell, McColl, Polatajko, & Pollock, 1998) was the tool used during the first meeting between Lisa and the occupational therapist. Lisa narrated her story while Rena, the occupational therapist, recorded the occupational areas of concern (OPIs) on the COPM. Once Lisa had finished her story, Rena paraphrased and summarized the OPIs identified, and Lisa validated all but one OPI as correct. This one was discussed until it was restated satisfactorily. Lisa then went back through the issues and rated them in terms of importance (on a scale of 1 to 10) on the COPM, thus prioritizing them. With each of the issues now identified and prioritized, Lisa then rated her current performance (on a scale of 1 to 10) and her current satisfaction (on a scale of 1 to 10) related to each of these issues on the COPM. Thus, Stage 1 of the OPPM has been completed with focus on occupation; identification of unique OPIs through narration, validation, and prioritization of those issues; and the initiation of outcome measures.

In Lisa's case, it looked like this:

> *I came into the hospital 2 days ago. I'm really a wreck, and I don't know how I'm ever going to cope when I go home. My mother is helping out right now but she has commitments she has to return to within 2 weeks, and she lives about a 5-hour drive from us. I feel like such a failure. I used to cope so well, balancing the demands of my work life with my home life. So much has changed during this pregnancy and since my second child arrived. We moved into a new house 6 months ago because we felt we needed the extra space. My husband works as a contractor and has been working as many jobs as he can to pay for the house. He's gone day and night, and, when he is home, he's returning phone calls or working on the books.*
>
> *I think the trouble started before the baby was born. I worked up until 2 weeks before the delivery and juggled my daughter back and forth to daycare. When I wasn't working, I was unpacking and trying to set up the new house. My daughter is 2, so she's into everything. I felt exhausted even before my son arrived. When Justin was born, he had some trouble feeding initially, and I can remember thinking "I just can't handle this!" I started to detach. I would look at him and think he is my baby and I love him, but I didn't feel anything. When I got home, things really fell apart. The baby was feeding every 3 hours, and my daughter started getting up through the night, too. I wasn't able to sleep much myself. Before long, I wasn't responding to anything. I often didn't shower for days, I had to force myself to make simple meals for my daughter, laundry was stacking up, and I felt helpless when the baby cried because I didn't know what to do to soothe him.*
>
> *I felt so bad, and my daughter, Kelly, didn't understand. She wanted me to play with her. Her schedule had changed, too. We were both home more, and she wanted my continual attention. I kept saying "Not now...I'm tired" or "I'm not feeling well." After a few days of these excuses, she started to scream or yell to get my attention, often waking the baby.*

It all came to a head last Friday when a neighbor dropped in and had to call my husband home from work. I was curled up in a corner. I was so depressed and anxious I could barely get words out. My daughter had been eating from the box of cereal I had left out for her, and the baby had been crying for what seemed like hours. Dirty dishes from the day before lined the kitchen, and I just wanted out.

I feel a bit better since I've come into hospital, but I'm frightened that the same thing will happen if I return home. I don't want to let everyone down again, and I'm worried that I can't be a good mother to my children. My husband, Tom, has been in visiting with the kids, and I genuinely feel happy to see them, but I am filled with guilt. Tom and my mom have been great supports, but I can tell they are frightened, too. I really worry about Tom in particular. He has a lot on the go, and he looks so stressed out. When I think about the things I have ahead of me, like getting back to work in 6 months, I feel hopeless and overwhelmed.

Rena empathetically supported Lisa's feelings and affirmed the numerous changes and increased demands she had undergone in the past 6 months. She summarized the occupational concerns (OPIs) identified in Lisa's story and asked her to confirm whether or not they were valid.

- Lisa felt confused, taking more than 20 minutes to respond to baby Justin's cries for food, hygiene, and nurturing.
- Kelly frequently roamed the house unsupervised, without diaper changes, until Tom came home.
- Lisa is struggling with basic child care and is unable to supervise Kelly's safety or provide stimulating play opportunities.
- Difficulty sleeping after the children are settled at night (on average only attaining 2 hours of sleep per night).
- Lisa's schedule of personal hygiene was reduced to showers once a week.
- Lisa felt overwhelmed with household demands (cleaning and organization, laundry, meal preparation, and shopping) and unable to engage in these activities and balance them with child care demands.

Lisa validated the above list of OPIs as being representative of her current concerns. She then put them in order of importance and rated her present performance and satisfaction with each of these issues on the COPM (Table 10-1).

Stage 1 of the OPPM is now complete. Lisa has had an opportunity to tell her story, and it has been confirmed that many of the issues are occupational in nature. Lisa and Rena are in agreement regarding the concerns that will be addressed, and these occupationally based issues have been measured pre-intervention using the COPM.

Table 10-1
Pre-Intervention Measurement of OPIs Using the COPM

OPI	Importance (1=not important, 10=very important)	Performance (1=not able to do it, 10=able to do it very well)	Satisfaction (1=not satisfied, 10=very satisfied)
Lisa felt confused, taking more than 20 minutes to respond to baby Justin's cries for food, hygiene, and nurturing.	10	2	1
Kelly frequently roamed the house unsupervised, without diaper changes, until Tom came home.	10	3	1
Lisa is struggling with basic child care and is unable to supervise Kelly's safety or provide stimulating play opportunities.	10	1	1
Difficulty sleeping after the children are settled at night (on average only attaining 2 hours of sleep per night).	9	3	2
Lisa's schedule of personal hygiene was reduced to showers once a week.	8	3	2
Lisa felt overwhelmed with household demands, unable to engage in these, and balance them with child care demands.	8	2	2

Total score = total performance or satisfaction scores / number of problems (COPM)
Performance 1: 14/6 = 2.3
Satisfaction 1: 9/6 = 1.5

Note: Please refer to the COPM manual for more information on scoring procedures.

Highlights of Stage 1

- Listen to client narration in context
- Focus on occupation
- Identify OPIs
- Validate and prioritize issues
- Evaluate occupational performance (OPIs) to create a baseline for use in outcome measurement

STAGE 2—SELECT THEORETICAL APPROACHES

Stages 1 and 2 of the OPPM actually have a large degree of overlap. As Lisa is telling her story in Stage 1, Rena attempts to make sense of these issues based on her understanding of occupational therapy theory. In this stage, Rena cogitates possible origins of these issues, testing these best guesses in Stage 3 through additional assessment and ultimately utilizing those confirmed theoretical approaches to drive intervention. This stage of the model is actually the therapist's thought process. Theory is one aspect of expertise the therapist brings to the client–therapist partnership. Hence, therapists can be encouraged to "name" selected theoretical models and use them to "frame" subsequent assessment and intervention. Occupational therapy theory provides a means of conceptualizing occupation and the aspects of people or environments that may affect occupational performance. Therefore, theoretical models considered may relate to aspects of occupation, person, or environment.

In Lisa's case, Rena considers psychological–emotional theories, specifically cognitive–behavioral approaches and physical and social environment theories.

Highlights of Stage 2

- Select potential theoretical approaches related to occupation, person, and environment as fit within the context of the client's story
- Select theoretical approaches to drive subsequent assessments and interventions

---

STAGE 3—IDENTIFY OCCUPATIONAL PERFORMANCE COMPONENTS AND CONDITIONS

Additional assessment is now completed to determine the possible components (person) or conditions (environment) contributing to the presenting OPIs (Canadian Association of Occupational Therapists, 1997). As it was Rena's speculation that Lisa's perception of events, expectations of self, and resulting depression and anxiety are contributing to Lisa's OPIs, she may seek subsequent data to support this. Suggested tools may be the Mind Over Mood Depression Inventory or the Mind Over Mood Anxiety Inventory (Greenberger & Padesky, 1995). To gather information about Lisa's occupations in the physical and social environments of her home and community settings, the Safety Assessment of Function and the Environment for Rehabilitation (SAFER) (Letts, Scott, Burtney, Marshall, & McKean, 1998) assessment tool is used.

Rena discussed the outcome of these assessments with Lisa, and she validated that the information represented a clear picture of her difficulties. These data were then compiled in a problem list and attributed to the related OPIs identified in Stage 1 (Table 10-2).

The left side of Lisa's problem list represents her OPIs, and the right side represents the personal components or conditions contributing to these issues. In terms of

---

Table 10-2
Problem List: Lisa's OPIs and Related Components and Conditions

OPI	Related Components or Conditions
Lisa felt confused, taking more than 20 minutes to respond to baby Justin's cries for food, hygiene, and nurturing.	• Lisa has a high frequency of self-depreciatory thoughts related to her role as a mother • Current means of dealing with anxiety is maladaptive (retreating to bed) • Fatigue • Lack of routine organization of tasks • Two-story house with bedrooms, changing areas, playroom, kitchen, laundry, and washrooms on three different floors
Kelly frequently roamed the house unsupervised, without diaper changes, until Tom came home.	• As per above
Lisa is struggling with basic child care and is unable to supervise Kelly's safety or provide stimulating play opportunities.	• As per above • Lisa lacks understanding of age-appropriate indoor/outdoor and quiet forms of play • Kelly's toys are not organized in appropriate settings that can be made secure and safe • Unaware of resources
Difficulty sleeping after the children are settled at night (on average only attaining 2 hours of sleep per night).	• Lisa ruminates during the night about the upcoming day • Unaware of "sleep induction" forms of relaxation
Lisa's schedule of personal hygiene was reduced to showers once a week.	• Lisa frequently leaves personal care routines for completion after child care activities. Due to demands, however, she rarely finds time to complete these tasks, and then does not wish to leave the house or have people come in, related to low images of self.
Lisa felt overwhelmed with household demands, unable to engage in these, and balance them with child care demands.	• Limited time • Lack of support and assistance • Lack of routine • Unaware of resources (e.g., grocery delivery)

documentation, occupational therapy notes on Lisa's chart now include the COPM, copies of the Depression and Anxiety Scales, the SAFER home visit assessment, and the problem list. This list of issues provides an analysis of all pertinent data and organizes the information in a manner that gives us some idea where to begin. Intervention will largely be directed at resolving barriers on the right side (components and conditions) of the problem list with implementation or adaptation in desired occupations.

Highlights of Stage 3

- Use additional assessments to investigate possible personal components or environmental conditions that may be contributing to the OPIs
- Observe relevant occupations in environments that make sense (context)
- Ensure assessments fit within the client's story
- Explain results of formal and informal assessment findings to clients through ongoing, jargon-free discussion
- Formulate and validate the problem list with the client

STAGE 4—IDENTIFY STRENGTHS AND RESOURCES

Rena asked Lisa about personal strengths that she felt might be helpful in the resolution of issues, and together they reviewed resources that may prove beneficial to the plan.

Lisa's personal strengths:
- Motivated to provide "best" parenting
- Creativity
- Enjoys social interaction and is now prepared to ask for help

Resources:
- Supported by mother, husband, extended family, neighbors, and friends
- One neighbor is an experienced mother of young children
- Lisa's sister-in-law is a pre-school teacher
- Lisa has access to many infant/tot services and programs through her community center and local public health unit
- Babysitting services exist within the neighborhood and community
- Funds may exist within the family budget to support assistance with household maintenance once per week
- The local grocery store provides online service with free delivery

Highlights of Stage 4

- Use formal and informal tools to gather information regarding client strengths in person and occupation and resources in his or her environment
- Consider the strengths and resources therapists bring to the client-therapist partnership
- Consider whether the therapist has the necessary knowledge and skill to positively influence change
- Integrate this information into the intervention plan as appropriate

STAGE 5—NEGOTIATE TARGETED OUTCOMES AND DEVELOP ACTION PLANS

Typically, each OPI identified will have a targeted outcome (goal) and an action plan (intervention or means of getting there) developed in this stage. For the purpose of this example, one of Lisa's OPIs will be used to develop a targeted outcome and related action plan.

OPI: Lisa is struggling with basic child care and is unable to supervise Kelly's safety or provide stimulating play opportunities.

Targeted Outcome: The targeted outcome is Lisa's vision of the future related to the above-mentioned OPI. Rena and Lisa have stated this outcome in behavioral terms, and Lisa has assigned a time frame she feels is reasonable in order to measure progress. Lisa's targeted outcome was: "Within 1 week, Tom and I will set up play environments for Kelly in our home where she may safely play independently for up to 10 minutes. Within 2 weeks, I will engage in play/stimulation activities with Kelly and Justin for up to 2 hours per day."

Action Plan: The action plan is directly related to the components and conditions Lisa identified in Stage 3 as barriers to her ability to supervise and play with Kelly. Through intervention, Rena and Lisa will first focus on the resolution of the contributing factors in person. Secondly, environmental adaptation or enhancements are made. Finally, Lisa will begin a graded return to her occupational context (Law, Cooper, Strong, Stewart, Rigby, & Letts, 1996). While weaving in Lisa's strengths and resources, Stage 5 of the OPPM constitutes the "what" and "who" of the intervention plan. Each item identified is explained, negotiated, and confirmed with Lisa. Partners and alliances are also identified and confirmed. Time frames are assigned for achievement of each step of the plan. The action plan for this targeted outcome is:

(Person)

1. Cognitive therapy—To decrease self-deprecating statements as measured in Mind Over Mood Depression Inventory (to be completed with the occupational therapist within 1 to 2 days).
2. Relaxation techniques—To include one form of "active" relaxation and one form of "deep" relaxation, particularly "sleep induction," in daily routine (to be completed with the occupational therapist within 3 to 4 days).
3. Lisa will expand her awareness of age-appropriate indoor/outdoor and quiet play activities for Justin and Kelly using her sister-in-law as a resource (to be completed in 2 to 3 days).

(Environment)

1. With the help of husband, mother, sister-in-law, and neighbor, Lisa will centralize a safe play area for Kelly and changing/feeding area for Justin on the main floor of the house, allowing Lisa to observe Kelly's play while engaged in Justin's care. Sleep areas will remain on the second floor with the use of baby monitors. Cupboards or containers of toys and supplies will be organized for both children, providing easy access for daily play and stimulation (to be completed in 3 to 5 days).
2. Lisa will join a mother and tot program at the community center and make use of the babysitting service there for Justin (to be completed in 5 to 7 days).

		Table 10-3	
	Documentation of Targeted Outcomes and Action Plans		
OPI	Related Components and Conditions	Intervention Plan	Date Resolved
		Targeted outcome: Action plan:	

3. Lisa and her neighbor (who also has a pre-school-aged child at home) will make arrangements for the children to play together every other day for periods up to 2 hours. Lisa will supervise and engage in this play in her home on alternate sessions (to be set up within 7 days).

(Occupation)

1. Lisa will develop a routine of personal care and child care tasks that may be somewhat flexible in nature and based on the routine or current demands of Justin's care. These activities will then be prioritized such that Lisa is able to engage in high priority occupations as time permits (a reasonable schedule of tasks to be completed in 3 to 4 days, Lisa will initiate practice with these routines on passes home within 5 days).
2. Lisa will engage in 30 minutes of play with Kelly (incorporating the above-mentioned skills, arrangements, and adaptations) within 5 days. She will add 5 minutes to this each day afterward until she has reached her target.
3. Lisa will also choose one replenishing occupation to engage in (creative or social) while the children are in the care of her husband (to be completed within 10 days).

With the action plan and targeted outcome now clearly in place, Lisa is eager to get started. Rena documents Lisa's targeted outcome and action plan for each of the OPIs she identified by adding a third column to the problem list (Table 10-3) titled "Intervention Plan." A fourth column, titled "Date Resolved," indicates when each issue is resolved, providing evidence that Lisa is making progress.

Highlights of Stage 5

- Determine the client's targeted outcome or vision of desired future performance related to OPIs
- Set targeted outcomes for each OPI
- Write targeted outcomes in behavioral terms and assign time frames for purposes of measurement
- Develop action plans based on all possible interventions in person, environment, and occupation that may positively influence the outcome
- Explain and negotiate interventions with clients
- Place the "what" of the action plan in order of necessary accomplishment with interventions in person generally first; then determine partnerships or the "who" of the plan and assign time frames

---

STAGE 6—IMPLEMENT PLANS THROUGH OCCUPATION

Rena made a copy of the plan for Lisa and her family, and all parties began fine-tuning the details, determining exactly "when" and "where" each step would take place. Rena and Lisa began cognitive therapy, and within three sessions Lisa was able to successfully challenge and reframe self-defeating thoughts. She began daily attendance at inpatient relaxation groups in the occupational therapy department and found active forms of relaxation a personal fit given her demanding lifestyle.

On the third day, Lisa began daily visits home of 1- to 3-hours duration. Her husband, Tom, and the neighbor initiated changes to the physical environment to facilitate ease of supervision, child care, and play, with Lisa's input. Lisa's sister-in-law was sick for a few days, but, by the first weekend home, she was able to meet with Lisa and Tom to help them set up toys and equipment that were age-appropriate for Kelly in a safe and stimulating environment. She also helped Lisa develop a list of activities she and Kelly could engage in at home.

Early the following week, Lisa and Tom took the children to a swimming program together and made the commitment to continue this once per week. Lisa also attended a mother and tot group at the community center. Lisa's mother went with them the first time to provide assistance with the children and moral support for Lisa. Kelly and Lisa enjoyed the active playtime in the gym. Lisa found conversation with the other parents not only stimulating but also validating and the child care for Justin more than satisfactory.

After a home visit, Rena made a number of recommendations based on a task analysis of the daily routine. With this information, Lisa and Tom then negotiated a daily schedule with which they both felt comfortable. Tom retired early in the evening, then woke early in the morning to feed Justin and put him back to sleep. Lisa rose, showered, dressed, and had breakfast with Tom before he left to work. This system would generally allow Lisa 45 minutes to an hour to prepare Kelly's breakfast and complete a few preparatory tasks for the day. As Lisa often felt most anxious and overwhelmed in the mornings, having an opportunity to engage in her active relaxation while doing these quiet tasks went a long way toward setting her day up for success. Lisa and Tom practiced this delineation of tasks before Lisa's discharge. Lisa's mother also agreed to stay with Lisa and Tom through this transition home, with a plan to gradually reduce her involvement in keeping with Lisa's comfort level.

In the progress notes section of Lisa's chart, Rena routinely documented achievement related to the plan. Each of these notes referred to the related OPI from the problem list. As each step of the action plan was completed, the date was noted under the column "Date Resolved." Progress notes and monitoring of accomplished steps of the plan continued until all had been completed and Lisa had attained her targeted outcome.

At the time of Lisa's discharge, she felt very positive about her increased performance in child care occupations. Everything appeared to be in place at home, and she was looking forward to weekly visits with friends. She discussed with Rena and other team members some of her outstanding concerns regarding possible relapse. It was decided that a referral would be made to community-based occupational therapy services where Lisa and a different therapist could revisit appropriate stages of the OPPM to address outstanding or recurring issues. It was also agreed that Lisa and her family would contact this resource if subsequent support was required.

Highlights of Stage 6

- Confirm the "when," "where," and "how" of the plan with all parties and begin the intervention
- Monitor and document progress
- Problem-solve possible lack of progress in partnership with the client, keep in mind the balance between content and process in this intervention phase, and be flexible
- Celebrate success and support grief related to potential frustration, fear, or loss
- Facilitate seamless transition of clients and documentation to other settings for continuation of the plan as required

---

STAGE 7—EVALUATE OCCUPATIONAL PERFORMANCE OUTCOMES

At the time of discharge, Lisa had achieved all of her targeted outcomes related to child care, personal hygiene, and household maintenance. She continued to experience some difficulty with sleep and planned to practice sleep induction relaxation techniques and follow-up with her family doctor. Rena and Lisa went back through the COPM to rescore her performance and satisfaction on the six OPIs she had originally identified (Table 10-4).

Lisa and her husband, Tom, were thrilled with her progress. They thanked Rena for the assistance occupational therapy provided and credited the rapid progress to the indi-

Table 10-4
Outcome Measurement of Lisa's OPIs Using the COPM

OPI	Performance Score 1 (pre-)	Performance Score 2 (post-)	Satisfaction Score 1 (pre-)	Satisfaction Score 2 (post-)
Lisa felt confused, taking more than 20 minutes to respond to baby Justin's cries for food, hygiene, and nurturing.	2	8	1	9
Kelly frequently roamed the house unsupervised, without diaper changes, until Tom came home.	3	8	1	9
Lisa is struggling with basic child care and is unable to supervise Kelly's safety or provide stimulating play opportunities.	1	9	1	10
Difficulty sleeping after the children are settled at night (on average only attaining 2 hours of sleep per night).	3	6	2	7
Lisa's schedule of personal hygiene was reduced to showers once a week.	3	8	2	8
Lisa felt overwhelmed with household demands, unable to engage in these, and balance them with child care demands.	2	7	2	8
Total change	14/6 = 2.3	46/6 = 7.6	9/6 = 1.5	51/6 = 8.5

vidualized and clearly articulated plan. Once home, Lisa, her family, and friends all commented on how helpful and empowered they felt throughout the process.

Rena completed the documentation on Lisa's chart by adding the outcome measures to the occupational therapy discharge summary. She also added these individualized outcomes to a data bank (averaged client outcomes) for program outcome purposes and justification of the service.

Highlights of Stage 7

- Measure client-specific targeted outcomes that are based in occupation
- Compare pre- and post-intervention measures
- Modify targets or identify additional goal areas as required
- Use individualized client outcomes collectively for program outcomes
- Use formal, reliable, and valid outcome measurement tools to provide the most useful information
- Use outcome measurement tools that make sense to stakeholders and are user-friendly for clients and therapists alike

---

As outlined in this case study, the OPPM provides a thorough and client-centered guideline for occupational therapy, whereby client momentum is reinstated. From the identification of issues through intervention to the measurement of outcomes, the process remains based in the client's individual context. In addition to guiding the therapy process, the OPPM may also be used to organize documentation, supporting data and tools in each of the seven stages. Chapter 11 will consider additional applications of the OPPM.

REFERENCES

Canadian Association of Occupational Therapists (CAOT) (1997). *Enabling occupation: An occupational therapy perspective*. Ottawa, Ontario, Canada: CAOT Publications ACE.

Fearing, V.G., Law, M., & Clark, J. (1997). An occupational performance process model: Fostering client and therapist alliances. *Canadian Journal of Occupational Therapy, 64*, 7-15.

Greenberger, D., & Padesky, C. (1995). *Mind over mood*. New York: Guilford Press.

Law, M., Baptiste, S., Carswell, A., McColl, M.A., Polatajko, H., & Pollock, N. (1998). *Canadian Occupational Performance Measure (COPM)* (3rd ed.). Ottawa, Ontario, Canada: CAOT Publications.

Law, M., Cooper, B., Strong, S., Stewart, D., Rigby, P., & Letts, L. (1996). The Person-Environment-Occupation model: A transactive approach to occupational performance. *Canadian Journal of Occupational Therapy, 63*, 9-23.

Letts, L., Scott, S., Burtney, J., Marshall, L., & McKean, M. (1998). The reliability and validity of the Safety Assessment of Function and the Environment for Rehabilitation (SAFER tool). *British Journal of Occupational Therapy, 61*, 127-132.

chapter eleven

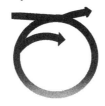

APPLICATIONS: THE PROCESS MODEL AS CATALYST FOR CHANGE

VIRGINIA G. FEARING, BSc(OT), OT(C), OTR,
Jo CLARK, BSc(OT), OT(C)

When you begin to use the Occupational Performance Process Model (OPPM) (Fearing, Clark, & Stanton, 1998), you may find that it alters the way you are used to practicing. If so, you are not alone. Many of us who use the OPPM have had to come to terms with the results of a true client-centered approach. First, we learned a new or different way of being with clients. We discovered that when it comes to being able to use theory, we could not get away with being "Johnny one note." It might be comfortable for us to view the world through our familiar approach (perhaps psycho-emotional), but we soon learned that our personal approach is not always what the client requires. Thus, therapists who had specialized began the process of broadening their horizons while maintaining their specialty.

Then we learned that when we stay with clients through the whole process of problem resolution, we are forced to address barriers to their function. This resulted in both frightening and exhilarating experiences, as we began to become true client advocates. We are learning how to take necessary risks without alienating everyone around us. We have made mistakes as we learn how to take on a whole organization over issues that matter, and we have learned from those mistakes. In short, now that our client-centered values are brought alive through a client-centered process, we are discovering the power of **bold** and **clear** messages based on values we live. It takes a while to adapt, but it usually doesn't take long for this approach to become second nature, mostly because it is so rewarding.

Because you are skilled at problem-solving, it won't take you long to identify the points of friction between a client-centered practice and the systems that are supposed to support that practice. We found that the systems we were used to, and had often created ourselves, were no longer useful. Thus began the next round of changes as we started to alter or develop systems to support our practice.

In this chapter, we share with you some of the changes we have made as a direct result of using the OPPM. Our purpose is to encourage you to change systems to support client-centered practice rather than changing practice to support systems. Adopt anything we share here in your own practice, if you wish, and adapt it to fit your own needs. When you are comfortable using the OPPM, we encourage you to explore how to change systems to support your own practice. No doubt you will develop innovative solutions of your own. We look forward to hearing about what you develop and also to seeing how others continue developing the approaches we use.

PROGRAM DESIGN: FIT OR MISFIT

As we focus on resolving specific client issues, it soon becomes clear when currently available programs do not meet client needs. To be blunt, we found that we had been plugging clients into programs because the programs were there, not because they promoted resolution of client issues. We could see that this was not good practice. So we developed a program design process (Appendix A), which we have found to be very useful in supporting client-centered practice.

Programs that do not meet client needs are a source of frustration and a poor investment of time for clients and therapists alike. We know that programs are a just right fit when clients not only take responsibility, but also are excited and committed to the process. Indicators that services may not fit include individuals not attending, being resistive to involvement, not following-up on recommendations, and therapists labeling clients as "unmotivated" or "uncooperative."

It helps clients to resolve the issues that are important to them if they are in a program that is designed to enable that resolution. This means that programs are designed with specific populations in mind. How do we know what issues this population generally wants to resolve? We do a needs assessment. First of all, we determine whether or not the target population has occupational performance issues (OPIs). If not, program development stops.

If the population surveyed does have OPIs, we review those OPIs to look for similarities and differences. If we are reviewing a program that is already in place, the needs assessment is easy, because all we have to do is keep a record of the OPIs that current clients are identifying. If a program is not in place and the intention is to design a new program, collect information from a number of individuals who are representative of the targeted population. Ensure that enough people are surveyed to result in useful data. The Canadian Occupational Performance Measure (Law, Baptiste, Carswell, McColl, Polatajko, & Pollock, 1998) may be used to gather information related to occupational performance. This is an especially effective method, as the results will be individualized. Over a period of time, data can be ranked in a table similar to Table 11-1.

It is important to understand similarities in issues associated with people, their environments, and their occupations. This gives us valuable information on which to base the design of the program. Using the data in Table 11-1 as an example, we may decide that when more than 70% of those surveyed share an OPI, we have reason to develop a program. This does not mean that we will neglect OPIs that are not shared by most of those surveyed, as these issues may be dealt with on an individualized basis. Sometimes we are

---

Table 11-1
Frequency of OPIs, Components, and Conditions

OPIs		Components and Conditions Contributing to OPIs	
Meal preparation	87%	Fatigue	94%
Mobility in the community	83%	Muscle strength compromised	90%
Return to work issues	46%	Accommodation not accessible	88%
Ability to dress and bathe	42%	Perceptual motor difficulties	88%
Parenting issues with young		Limited standing tolerance	82%
children	39%	Visual deficits	48%
Ability to resume active leisure	35%		

---

able to develop a program flexible enough to meet those needs, too. Usually, we focus program development on issues that are shared by many. The challenge is to develop a program that has program outcomes while at the same time enabling achievement of individual outcomes. That is, the program is cohesive enough to meet the needs of a group of people, yet flexible enough to meet the needs of individuals within the group.

We know we have succeeded when clients enrolled in the program resolve OPIs that are important to them. Programs or services that are designed around client-specific occupations look completely different from those that focus on components or parts of the body. For this reason, the program design format (see Appendix A) is designed to force the user to identify expected client occupational performance outcomes as a result of this program. Our experience is that therapists want to record that the outcome will be that clients are assessed and that they are treated. This is not a client-expected outcome, but rather therapist process. It can be helpful to ask "So what?" So what if they are assessed? So what if they are treated? Then, we may get something like, so clients will be as independent as possible. So what? Eventually, we get to a client-centered outcome. Identifying expected client outcomes seems to be the hardest part of the program design process. Once determined, however, the rest of program development is easy. We use this program design process to review current programs and to document proposed programs. This approach makes it clear which client outcomes will be purchased (or lost) with an increase (or decrease) in staff. It is much easier to "sell" a program based on client outcomes than on therapist interventions or workload, although of course we know they are related. We have effectively used this method to maintain and promote staffing levels.

Given the constant change in people, the environments we live in, and the resources around us, the need to routinely review our services prevails. Such review can be ongoing or completed at predetermined intervals and carried out in different ways. We can compare the issues identified in Stage 1 of the OPPM with the outcomes in Stage 7. What matters to clients is whether or not their priority issues are resolved. If we discover absence of resolution or movement on client priority issues, it is important to understand why. If issues are not resolved, it can be revealing to track back through the process. That is, compare issues identified in Stage 1 with interventions used in Stage 6. What is done in Stage 6 should support resolution of issues and therefore needs to make sense in relation to both the issues identified as priority in Stage 1 and also the expected outcomes evaluated in Stage 7. If it doesn't make sense, why doesn't it? If it does make sense, what is working? Reviewing interventions planned in Stage 5, and especially whether or not they address OPIs, can suggest program connect or disconnect with clients. What do clients think? It is important to ask clients what meaning the program has for them. When the process happens as it should, we expect to see high levels of success in our outcome measures for each client individually, as well as for the program as a whole. At times, services or interventions continue as they always have simply as a matter of history. However, being placed in a program that doesn't fit can be as painful in its own way as cramming a foot into the only shoe available, regardless of the fit. Misfits hurt. Fit enables function.

SELF-REFERRAL:
I HAVE A BRAIN AND I WOULD LIKE TO USE IT

Refer means "To send or direct for treatment, aid, information, decision" (*Webster's*, 1981, p. 1907). In some cases, law regulates referral to occupational therapy. In these cases, someone else, usually a physician, serves as the gatekeeper to client access to occupational therapy practice. Where access is not regulated by law or organizational rules, occupational therapists may choose to institute a client self-referral process, which assists the client to identify priority OPIs that matter enough to seek assistance from an occupational therapist. Wilson (1999) has developed and is successfully using a client self-referral process that assists clients to screen for their own OPIs and to refer themselves. As well as serving as a tool for clients, the self-referral form has the potential to assist physicians, and others, to screen more accurately.

As client priority issues are resolved and recorded in a way that has meaning to clients and others, word about occupational therapy spreads. Resolution of client issues is the most effective marketing tool we will ever have. As clients and colleagues see the results of a practice focused on resolving issues, referrals may increase, resulting in increased workload. Concern that client self-referral might lead to an increased workload is better addressed through workload management than denying clients access.

PRIORITY INTERVENTION CRITERIA:
WHOSE PRIORITY? WHAT CRITERIA?

A surprising number of therapists have reported to the first author that all they have time to do, given current caseloads, is to assess and move on to the next client, in this way never getting beyond assessment. A focus on client outcomes will require re-evaluation of this practice. Seeing half of the clients but remaining with them through resolution or planned resolution of their issues is far more effective than identifying all the issues and the components and conditions contributing to them and resolving none.

Because the demands of clinical caseloads often exceed existing resources, wait lists are generated, indicating the need for some kind of system to prioritize those referred to the service. We have been experimenting with a Priority Intervention Criteria (PIC) system as a method to assist us in collaborative and objective priority setting (Rackow, 1996). The principle is that we all set priorities within our own minds and act on those priorities, although we often don't share them with others. As a result, we may find ourselves judging, or being judged by others, because we do not meet each other's (unnamed) expectations.

The process of developing a PIC is to gather colleagues working in the same area and come to agreement regarding what will be considered priority issues. The criteria used will need to be determined. For example, the criteria may be safety, time to discharge, or potential for prevention of admission to a facility. Whatever are chosen as criteria are then ranked. If prevention is chosen as the criterion, can we agree on what Priority 1 would be? That is, of all the clients referred to your service for prevention of OPIs, which ones will have priority, those at greatest risk or those with the most potential to learn quickly?

As each person shares the criteria he or she uses to determine priority, the group gains insight into why others are practicing as they do. It may take a while to achieve consensus, however, it is worth coming to agreement. The challenge in developing a priority intervention system is to select a framework that makes sense in that particular setting. For example, a system that is time-based might mean that OPIs that must be addressed within 24 hours would be PIC 1. If they can wait a week, they may be PIC 3. Perhaps you will decide that resolution of OPIs that are most costly to the funding agent have priority. Whatever system is developed, the fact that it is organized and based on a group decision makes it far easier to share heavy workloads.

Our experience is that the current pressure to discharge clients quickly means a more rapid "through-put" of clients in acute and rehabilitation care with clients returning to the community in a more fragile state. As a result, therapists in facilities are no longer able to address lower priorities. This is useful information during budget discussions. A cut in funding 2 years ago might have resulted in reduced resolution of OPIs at low priority levels. Today, a cut in funding might result in reduced resolution of priority issues, thus affecting the cost efficiency of the funding agent. Whatever the priority scale, once the criterion is set, therapists screen clients for OPIs and meet regularly to sort referrals into priority levels. Assignments can be developed for daily or weekly caseloads, although therapists manage the sharing of caseloads very well given this systematic approach and demonstrate flexibility should new priorities suddenly develop. PIC helps to clarify expectations and make caseloads explicit. Staff report that it also decreases feelings of guilt for work not done because it is more obvious what it is possible to do.

Whose priorities are we serving? If we base our PIC on OPIs identified by clients, then we are serving client priorities. When we communicate clearly to clients and funding agencies the types of issues that will have priority, then, although people may argue about the criteria, they cannot fault the fairness. Therapists tend to find it very hard to slow down enough to be present with a client, knowing that other clients are not being seen. However, a shared decision to make a difference to a few rather than briefly interacting with the many serves some clients well.

The primary recipients of the pressures exerted on the health care system continue to be the clients. This pressure flows over onto therapists who work to adapt to changing and escalating demands. This can result in heavy workloads and therapists too busy to step back and think about what is happening. The easiest response to heavy workload is to cry for more staff. This approach is usually based on therapist overwork and need. This is not always successful, as it is common to wonder if the service is as efficient as it could be. Another approach is to collect PIC data for a period of time and develop a program design that addresses unmet needs in such a way that the focus is on potential client outcomes given program support.

EXPERIENCE, EXPERTISE, AND CONTINUITY OF CARE

While students and most therapists learn to use the OPPM with ease, some experienced therapists find it very difficult to move from a focus on components to a focus on client OPIs and the components contributing to those issues. Their valuable knowledge regarding components could be so much more effective if it was connected to client priority issues. Many students and newly graduated therapists find it difficult to focus on components without understanding their relationship to OPIs. When different therapists use similar approaches, the OPPM can contribute to continuity of care. Because the OPPM is client-based and not therapist-based, the process may be started in one setting, continued in another, and completed in still another. In these cases, client issues may be identified in one setting and resolved in another. This means that several different therapists may be involved in enabling resolution of issues important to the client.

STANDARDS OF PRACTICE

Key standards of practice may be used to promote and support client-centered practice. Appendix B is an example of a health record standard of practice currently in use. These particular standards are compatible with the parent organization's interdisciplinary standards of documentation and have assisted occupational therapists in securing a vital place for client occupational performance function in the interdisciplinary health record. The Profile of Occupational Therapy Practice in Canada (Canadian Association of Occupational Therapists, 1996) may be used as a basis for developing practice standards that support each stage of the OPPM, however, it is important to maintain the flow of the occupational performance process as a whole, rather than over-focus on parts.

The health, or professional, record of service has the potential to become a tool that assists clinical reasoning as well as documents the service that is provided (Fearing, 1993). Because many occupational therapists work within a team setting, it may be necessary to adapt current methods of using forms to be able to record client priority issues, targeted and achieved outcomes, and plans to achieve those outcomes. While it is important to meet legal and organizational requirements for documentation, concise and focused documentation is an art that is appreciated by all those who read it. Therapists, who reflect on the meaning of what they write, document so that the client may comfortably view the health record. They report in behavioral language only that which is pertinent to the current episode.

HUMAN RESOURCES: THE RIGHT PEOPLE IN THE RIGHT PLACE HAVING A GREAT TIME

In order to implement a client-centered approach to practice, it is important to carefully select therapists who are healthy within themselves and whose behaviors reflect an enabling approach to being with others. It helps to have clearly articulated job descriptions that identify at the very least the core competencies that are required. Recruitment is clearly an important part of creating a client-centered service. Interestingly, we have found that creating a client-centered service has helped with recruitment.

Recently, we have begun experimenting with hiring people whose values are congruent with a client-centered approach. That is, we realized that we can teach people skills but we cannot teach them values. So our interview process explores what the applicants are really passionate about in occupational therapy. What approach do applicants take and can be expected to take regarding continuing education? What is the most interesting journal article they have read recently? What do they have to say about the theoretical approaches they are comfortable using? How do they bring client-centered practice alive in their everyday work, and what behaviors could we expect to see them exhibit in their practice? This has led to lively and engaging discussion on the one hand and effective selection on the other. It does not mean that all people hired should be alike. On the contrary, a rich mix of staff contributes to a healthy environment as long as key, core values are shared.

We are open about our expectation that staff provide leadership in their everyday practice by enabling others (clients, families, and team and committee members) to be the people they want to be while at the same time remaining true to their own values (see Chapters 1 and 2). We talk about our vision for research and our vision for education. And finally, although not least importantly, we try in one way or another to convey that ours is an environment where it is okay to laugh, to celebrate, and to take the risk of trying new ways. The process of hiring, orienting, and developing staff to behaviors and expectations that support a healthy environment and client-centered practice contributes to building continuous learning as the norm.

PERFORMANCE APPRAISAL: AM I JUMPING HIGH ENOUGH?

Performance appraisal is a process that includes surveying others and conveying the resulting information (usually in an anonymous aggregate) to the subject. This process answers the question: "Am I jumping high enough?" This is only as humane as the people involved and, even so, is dependent on each person's values and expectations. When the feedback is anonymous, it loses effectiveness because we do not know the context from which the feedback comes. That is, if the subject is a research scientist and a reviewer does not value or understand research, the subject will not be able to place the review comments in context.

A focus on performance development instead of performance appraisal can shift the emphasis to what to learn next. This answers the question: "How can I learn to do a twist and a half while I jump?" At some point, the subject will complain that there is no point in another performance appraisal because the limits of the jump have been reached.

The question that matters is "Am I reflecting on whether or not jumping serves a purpose and am I open to learning how to skip?" The Client-Centred Process Evaluation (CCPE) (see Chapter 13), combined with keeping a personal portfolio, has the potential to become an effective performance reflection approach. Am I jumping high enough? It depends on who's asking and who's answering, and whether jumping is the best thing to do.

VISIONS: IMAGINING AND CREATING A DESIRED FUTURE

Block (1987) reminds us that "Creating a vision forces us to take a stand for a preferred future." He continues by telling us that

> Not just any vision will do...The vision needs to be lofty in order to capture our imagination and engage our spirit. Inspired performance is characterized by a lofty vision...Our vision is our deepest expression of what we want. The vision works because only if others know what we want can they support us. It is the dialogue about vision that helps us connect with each other in a way that matters. (pp. 108-109)

The power of developing a vision for the future from a practice based in occupation was apparent when 16 occupational therapists, including those from each local site and from the university faculty, were able to develop a collaborative vision for research within 3 hours. The vision is as follows:

> At VHHSC, occupational therapists are dedicated to excellence in practice based on thoughtful reflection, participation in research, and publication of results. In partnership with the UBC academic faculty in the School of Rehabilitation Sciences, occupational therapists will gather evidence about occupational therapy practice that makes a difference to occupational performance that is valued by the client. (VHHSC, 1998)

One year after the vision was incorporated into a strategy for occupational therapy research, and thanks to support from the University and Vancouver Hospital, we are able to announce the impending arrival of an Occupational Therapy Research Scientist cross-appointed with the University as Assistant Professor. This electric development so galvanized us that we created a vision for education.

A different but representative group began working on developing a vision for education and a strategy to support it. The vision is: "Occupational therapists at VHHSC are committed to learning as a way of being."

LEARNING AS A WAY OF BEING: MENTORING AS A METHOD

When we are working to achieve a vision for our future, and particularly one that is well known by others, it is possible to explore different ways of getting there. In this case, staff have chosen to organize a full-day workshop focused on mentoring. One of the agreed-upon principles is that everyone is a mentor and everyone is an expert. The challenge is to make it safe for all staff, regardless of experience, to be both novice and expert at the same time. Developing this comfort is critical to creating an environment where clients, therapists, and students may both teach and learn.

CONCLUSION

We have shared a few applications of the OPPM not so much as examples of what to do but rather as examples of how it is possible to respond to the need to change. Unable to foresee the future, and realizing that change is constant (and not always rational), we are working toward creating a stable base for client-therapist interactions regardless of the organizational structure in vogue. Envisioning a future is important. The analogy that works for us is to think of a group of boats frozen into the ice of a river, unable to move. Nobody can move in an environment that is frozen. When change occurs and the ice breaks up, chaos occurs. We know we don't want to be in the boat that cries "Mayday, mayday." We know we don't want to be in the boat that complains while spinning in circles. We know we don't want to be in the boat that blames the weather, the boat, others. We understand that chaos provides an opportunity to reposition ourselves. So we want to be in the boat with people who know where they want to be when the river freezes again, and, as long as we agree on the destination, we are willing to paddle like the dickens to get there. We especially want to be in the boat where respect and fun are part of the journey.

REFERENCES

Block, P. (1987). *The empowered manager* (pp. 108-116). San Francisco: Jossey-Bass Publishers.

Canadian Association of Occupational Therapists (CAOT). (1996). Profile of occupational therapy practice in Canada. *Canadian Journal of Occupational Therapy, 63,* 79-113.

Fearing, V.G. (1993). Occupational therapists chart a course through the health record. *Canadian Journal of Occupational Therapy, 60,* 232-240.

Fearing, V.G., Clark, J., & Stanton, S. (1998). The client-centred occupational therapy process. In M. Law (Ed.), *Client-Centered Occupational Therapy.* Thorofare, NJ: SLACK Incorporated.

Law, M., Baptiste, S., Carswell, A., McColl, M.A., Polatajko, H., & Pollock, N. (1998). *Canadian Occupational Performance Measure (COPM)* (3rd ed.) Ottawa, Ontario, Canada: CAOT Publications.

Rackow, B. (1996). *Priority Intervention Criteria.* Unpublished raw data.

VHHSC (Vancouver Hospital & Health Sciences Center). (1998). A strategic plan for occupational therapy research: a partnership between VHHSC and the School of Rehabiliation Sciences. UBC, p. 3.

Webster's Third New International Dictionary of the English Language Unabridged. (1981). Springfield, MA: Merriam-Webster.

Wilson, M. (1999). Client self-referral: Starting the process right. *Occupational Therapy Now, January/February,* 22-24.

section three

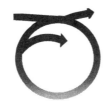

REFLECTING ON PRACTICE IN CONTEXT

chapter twelve

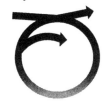

OPPORTUNITIES IN A CHANGING HEALTH CARE ENVIRONMENT

MARY J. BRIDLE, MA, OTR/L, OT(C), FAOTA,
CYNTHIA A. STABENOW, MS, OTR/L

> *The only constant is change.*
> (Schaef, 1996)

OVERVIEW

The client-therapist partnership occurs within the larger context of a changing health care environment. This chapter starts with some operational definitions followed by a discussion of some of the factors that drive change in health care environments. Organizational responses to such changes are briefly discussed along with their implications for the practitioner. Personal perceptions of and responses to change are addressed to enhance readers' awareness of their personal style in confronting change. Issues surrounding client-centered practice in the face of the challenges and constraints of today's health care environments are discussed, and some common concerns are addressed. Client self-advocacy is proposed, and strategies for facilitating it are discussed. Next, we consult our crystal ball for a look at the future and suggest possible new environments for occupational therapy. We close with a summary of the main points of the chapter.

JUST SO WE'RE ALL ON BOARD

The following terms are defined for the purpose of this chapter:

- A **health care provider** is the body that, or individual who, delivers and is remunerated for health care services. This may be an institution (e.g., hospital, clinic, etc.) or an individual health care professional such as you. Family members may provide care but they are not considered providers as the term is defined for this chapter.
- The **payer** is the institution or individual who pays for the health care services rendered. Payers may include Federal Governments, Provincial or State Governments, for-profit insurance companies, and clients. Some payers refer to themselves as providers because they pay the bills but, in this chapter, they are referred to as payers.

- The **clients** are the people to whom the services are delivered and/or their significant others or support personnel.
- The **health care environment** is the larger context of health care provision. It is country-specific and is affected by the local finances and politics.

CHANGE, PROGRESS, AND MONEY: MONEY TALKS

Change is constant. During this century, medical science and technology have changed extensively and rapidly. The discovery of disease causes and advances in pharmacology and surgical techniques underpin some of the greatest changes in health care in the 20th century. The discovery of insulin in 1922, penicillin in 1929, and the polio vaccine in 1955 combined to radically enhance life expectancy (Benson, 1997; Smith, 1990). Human organ transplantation was pioneered in the 1960s (Wythenshawe Hospital Manchester, 1999). Today, organ transplantation techniques and accompanying immunosuppressive therapies have developed to the point where organ transplantation is a common treatment option for some diseases. Joint replacement dates back to 1939 (Smyth, Freyberg, & McEwen, 1985). Currently, total joint replacement is widely used as the treatment of choice for people with painful, deteriorated joints.

We who live in Western countries reap the benefits of a century of change in medical care. We have an increase in the number of live births, a decrease in infant mortality, and an increase in life expectancy. We are able to effect cures, sustain life by artificial means, and postpone death. All this progress comes at a price. There are costs involved in bringing a troubled pregnancy to term and delivering a live child. Organ transplantation is an expensive option both in the short- and long-term. Our ability to sustain life through artificial means is another intervention that contributes to the overall increase in health care expenses.

The increase in life span is attributable to the improved sanitation, nutrition, and health care we have enjoyed in the 20th century. The average life expectancy in the United States increased from 47 years in 1900 to 72.3 for men and 79.1 for women in 1992 (Novartis Foundation, 1999). In Canada, people 65 and older are one of the fastest-growing segments of the population. Between 1981 and 1998, there was a 60% increase from 2.4 million to 3.7 million. This is projected to reach about 7 million in 2021 (Statistics Canada, 1997). The longer we live, the more likely we are to need health care and rehabilitation services for a variety of chronic diseases characteristic of the older population. Currently in the United States, there are 33.6 million persons age 65 or older. Americans age 85 and older represent the fastest growing segment of the population (Novartis Foundation, 1999). The bulge in the upper age group of the population brings an increased burden on the health care system. In Canada, the population aged 85 and older is growing faster than any other segment of the senior population (Statistics Canada, 1999). Lives are longer, but independence may not be preserved, thus, the cost of rehabilitation and long-term care increases. In 1990, in the United States, there were approximately seven million older people requiring long-term care. It is projected that this will rise to nine million by 2005 and 12 million in 2020 (Novartis Foundation, 1999). The trend is similar in Canada where 74% of all people living in institutions are 65 and older (Statistics Canada, 1999). Advances in medical care and increase in life expectancy impact occupational therapy as they increase the numbers of people requiring rehabilitation services.

Possibly the easiest way to appreciate the increase in health care costs is to look at the percent of the gross national product (GNP) that is spent on health care in a given year. In Canada, in 1976, health care expenditures were 7.1% of GNP and rose to 9.8% in 1994. In the following 2 years, it dropped to 9.6% in 1995 and 9.5% in 1996 (Health Canada, 1997). This modest decrease between 1994 and 1996 is the result of dramatic cuts in health care services as anyone who lives there can attest. Whether the trend continued through 1998 and 1999 is, as yet, unknown.

In the United States, health care expenditures were 5.2% of the GNP in 1960. By 1990, this figure was 12.2%, or $696.6 billion, and it is still rising. In the United States, health care spending will pass the trillion-dollar mark during 1999. The Health Care Financing Administration projects that the level could rise to 31.5% of the GNP in 2020 if current trends continue (Novartis Foundation, 1999).

Change begets change as payers and providers struggle to contain costs and, in some cases, maintain profits. In the next section, we shall look at the relationship between rising costs, policies, politics, and providers.

WAKE UP AND SMELL THE COFFEE: FINANCES AND POLITICS

Whether we realize it or not, all health care is financed by the population of a given country. Countries such as Canada and the United Kingdom have a single payer system, or "socialized medicine." Health care is financed through taxes. Everyone who pays taxes contributes to the health care of the entire population. The burden of the very sick is shared across the entire population. Administrative costs are less than those of a multiple payer system, simply because there is only one administration involved. Many of the developed countries of the world have a single payer system that ensures every citizen access to basic health care.

The system in the United States is an example of a multiple-payer system. The Federal Government provides health care to persons over 65 years of age and those persons considered too disabled to work through the Medicare program. State Governments provide for the very poor through the Medicaid program with funds provided by the Federal Government. Both these programs are paid for with tax dollars. Otherwise, health insurance is provided through private insurance companies. Typically, people who are employed full-time have health insurance provided as a fringe benefit. Those who are self-employed or employed part-time are responsible for acquiring their own insurance if they can afford it. Currently, about 45 million citizens in the United States are without any sort of health insurance, and the number is growing (American Occupational Therapy

Association, 1999). Neither the single-payer nor multiple-payer system is without disadvantage, and both are impacted by the rising cost of providing health care. In democratic countries, the system can be changed through political activism. Persons unhappy with their health care system need to be politically aware and active, because ultimately the politicians are involved in health care service decisions whatever the delivery system.

Payers try to control costs by limiting the number of health care visits allowed, policing provided services, requiring providers to justify services, and denying further care if improvement is not demonstrated. This can result in increased administrative costs for providers who, in turn, must find ways to provide effective service in less time at lower cost. Institutions may reorganize to reduce administrative costs. This may affect the chain of command, career ladders may be dismantled, salaries cut, positions eliminated, and personnel laid off. As a result, therapists may experience increased caseloads, restrictions on the number of therapy visits, increased documentation requirements, increased time spent justifying the need for therapy for individual clients, and fewer support staff. Change is, indeed, constant.

OF RUTS AND BOXES

Probably all of us are guilty of practicing in a rut at some time or other. Ruts are familiar and comfortable. Unfortunately, ruts foster limited thinking: "This is the way I do it" can become "This is the only way I can do it!" Our thinking is boxed in and our creativity stifled. Change threatens our ruts and boxes, and, though frightening, this can be a good thing.

How we perceive and respond to change dictates how we handle it. If we see it as a threat, we may respond angrily out of fear. If we perceive it as an enormous nuisance, we may respond grudgingly with hostility, and if we see it as an opportunity, we will likely respond with some enthusiasm and optimism.

Change is stressful because it demands that we climb out of our ruts and abandon our boxes. We may perceive change as a threat and respond with fear and resistance, as a challenge and rise to meet it, as an opportunity and exploit it. For many of us, this represents a continuum of reaction: first we resist; then, when we realize that's useless, we are able to view it as a challenge; and finally, we may be able to see that there are opportunities inherent in the change. The stress of change can become a catalyst for a client-centered practice. As therapists, we may not be responsible for the changes in the health care system, but we are responsible for helping our clients meet their goals within the confines of the new system. Together in partnership, you and the client can figure out how best to manage. Discussion of the client's priorities and goals can help clarify how and when limited therapy sessions should be used. When life hands you what looks like a lemon, make lemonade!

MAKING LEMONADE TOGETHER

In this section, we illustrate how to maintain a client-centered approach and meet client goals within the changing health care environment. The second author is responsible for providing occupational therapy in a skilled nursing facility (SNF). Most of her clients are covered by Medicare, which recently implemented draconian changes to the payment system, including limiting assessments to a maximum of 30 minutes. These changes require concurrent treatment and assessment and extreme efficiency on the part of the therapist.

The case of Mrs. D. illustrates the implementation of the Occupational Performance Process Model (Fearing, Clark, & Stanton, 1998) in the SNF environment. Mrs. D.'s payer selected the second author's facility as it offered the lowest daily rate for a package of therapy services, room, and board. The payer authorized 1500 minutes of therapy a week, for 2 weeks, to be divided among the three therapy services: occupational, physical, and speech therapy. Thus, the author had about 60 minutes a day, for 2 weeks, to provide an intensive occupational therapy program for Mrs. D. Previously, Medicare allowed 2 hours per day for 3 weeks or more at the therapist's discretion. Mrs. D. is 41 years old with a 20-year history of progressive multiple sclerosis. She is married and has a son. At the time of admission to the SNF, she had just finished a course of cytoxan infusion therapy and required rehabilitation before returning to her home.

STAGE 1—NAME, VALIDATE, AND PRIORITIZE OCCUPATIONAL PERFORMANCE ISSUES

Administration of the Canadian Occupational Performance Measure (Law, Baptiste, Carswell, McColl, Polatajko, & Pollock, 1994) helped Mrs. D. identify six occupational performance issues:

1. Limited ability to move around the house due to accessibility and fatigue issues
2. Inability to talk for more than 5 minutes without getting tired
3. Inability to go to the toilet in the early morning independently due to inability to walk and location of the bathroom
4. Inability to dress herself due to fatigue and poor balance
5. Lack of enjoyment of visits with relatives due to fatigue
6. Inability to use the computer to play games with her son for more than 5 minutes due to fatigue and accessibility issues

Due to space limitations here, resolution of the personal care issues only will be used to illustrate implementation of the model.

STAGE 2—SELECT POTENTIAL INTERVENTION MODELS

To address her personal care issues, physical-rehabilitative, neuro-integrative, and environmental approaches were the selected intervention models.

STAGE 3—IDENTIFY OCCUPATIONAL PERFORMANCE COMPONENTS AND ENVIRONMENTAL CONDITIONS

Mrs. D.'s problems with personal care were related to several components including fatigue, limited range of motion in her right shoulder, tremors in both hands, and instability in standing. Environmental conditions included the location of the bathroom relative to the bedroom and Mrs. D.'s dependence on her husband to carry her to the toilet in the early morning as she couldn't walk. Assessments included observation of her performing activities of daily living at the SNF and a home visit. Specific measures of range of motion, strength, and balance were left to physical therapy.

STAGE 4—IDENTIFY STRENGTHS AND RESOURCES

Mrs. D. was quick to point out that she has a very supportive husband and adequate financial resources. She has a personal care aide who comes every morning to assist with child care, meal preparation, and her personal care.

STAGE 5—NEGOTIATE TARGETED OUTCOMES AND DEVELOP ACTION PLANS

In particular, Mrs. D. wants to be able to go to the toilet and dress herself independently. The action plan was as follows: during a 2-week stay at the SNF, Mrs. D. will perform dressing and toileting with the caregiver present for three consecutive sessions by the end of the second week. The therapist will complete a home visit with Mrs. D. and her husband and recommend environmental modifications.

STAGE 6—IMPLEMENT PLANS THROUGH OCCUPATION

Mrs. D. was taught to use a bedside commode and used it independently every night during her stay in the SNF. She learned to select her clothing and put them on her walker at bedtime, and she was instructed in a safe dressing technique seated in a chair with arms. A home visit was completed during the second week of her SNF stay. Recommendations included the purchase of a bedside commode to permit independent toileting in the early morning, and the purchase of a sturdy shower transfer bench and a hand-held shower to ensure safety and a modicum of independence while showering with the assistance of her caregiver.

STAGE 7—EVALUATE OCCUPATIONAL PERFORMANCE OUTCOMES

Mrs. D. was satisfied with the resolution of her toileting and dressing performance problems.

The first author works in a freestanding, for-profit, outpatient therapy center. Clients are primarily adults. Many of them have acute hand injuries; others have acute or chronic repetitive strain injuries, many of which are work-related. Other clients have rheumatological diseases both newly diagnosed or long-standing. This practice has been affected by changes both in Medicare funding and private insurance. The beneficiaries are largely unaware of these changes so time must be spent explaining them to clients at the outset of therapy. Clients must understand that there are limits and be engaged in the decisions regarding how these visits will be used. Ironically, the new rules actually foster a client-centered approach.

Recent changes in Medicare legislation resulted in significant limits on the amount of outpatient therapy allowed in a calendar year. Private insurance companies have developed a variety of ways of controlling costs, one of which is managed care. Managed care requires that therapists obtain authorization for treatment. Therapists must make a good case in order to obtain treatment sessions, which are often meted out a few at a time. Payers want to know the goals of treatment and want to see measurable improvement before they will grant further sessions. If they are not convinced that progress is being made, they will not pay for further therapy. While this added bureaucracy increases the therapists' administrative burden, managed care can facilitate the client-centered approach. One client noted that knowing her insurance was limited was helpful in getting her motivated.

The changes that impact the daily practice of our profession call for flexibility and creativity. We need to be open to new ideas, and to review and revise how we think about things. We may need to revise our view of what a therapy session looks like. Therapists and clients have had to learn to tolerate frequent interruptions and to share time between two or more clients. While such changes may be upsetting to us, we need to remember that our clients may have a very different view.

Financial restraint evidences itself in a variety of ways. Budgets may not be cut but the number of clients to be served may be increased, which is the same thing in the end. We have to be able to do more with less. This is typical of changes in home health care funding both in Canada and the United States. In her article "Meeting the Challenge of New Home Health Care Mandates," Siebert (1999) demonstrates how occupational therapists and their home care clients can survive and even flourish by creatively adapting to the changes imposed from above. Together with our clients, we can define realistic priorities, be clear about how much therapy can contribute, and facilitate the client in finding ways of making up any shortfall.

The question may arise: "What if the client's priorities conflict with what the therapist thinks should be the priority?" If the therapist disagrees with the client's assessment of his or her problem, time needs to be spent investigating the nature of the disagreement. One thing is clear. If the therapy program is developed around priorities to which the client does not subscribe, a lot of time will be lost, and little progress will be made. We must take the time to understand the meaning of clients' problems and how to meet them despite restricted funding. One client put it very succinctly: "There is only one way of doing this, and that is my way." We did it his way, and he achieved his goals and was appreciative of the client-centered approach.

Another client of the first author came with a treatment program outlined by a therapist who lived on the other side of the country. The client was dedicated to the program approach and wished to continue, but the program did not make sense to the author.

After considerable discussion and explanation, agreement was reached, and a therapeutic alliance was formed. Had an understanding not been reached, the author would have said she could not work with the client. This is a difficult thing for occupational therapists to do because we are the world's greatest "fixers." We need to know when to hold and know when to fold.

Sometimes payers may be confused about who is the client. For example, in the case of an injured worker, the workers' compensation insurance carrier (payer) may think that it is the client. In fact, the client is the injured worker. Workers' compensation is an insurance policy bought and paid for by the employer and/or the employee. When workers are injured on the job, they are entitled to payment and medical and rehabilitation care as well as compensation for any residual functional losses. It may be necessary to enlighten the payer in this respect! Clients with workers' compensation are likely to have a case manager who is the gatekeeper and who may be torn between the client's priorities and those of the employer. Development of positive personal relationships with case managers is vital if we are to engage them in the clients' priorities. Conversely, a poor relationship between therapist and case manager will only harm the client.

The shift to client-centered practice may raise questions regarding how to convince payers to reimburse for therapy based on the client's priorities. We therapists are the interface between the client and payer, and our job is to represent the client as a person and not as a diagnosis with a claim number. We must become familiar with the payers' viewpoint and framework, we must understand the language they use, and we must use their language in our documentation. If there is any question about priorities or goals, we need to take the time to explain why it makes sense to follow the client's priorities. Sometimes it is helpful to do so in terms of money that can be saved or to protect an investment already made by the payer. For example, the first author had a client who had surgery to correct severe finger deformities caused by scleroderma. Subsequently, the client's fingers started contracting to their original position, and she required custom splints to prevent this from happening. Because her disease complicated the situation, the splinting was relatively expensive, and the insurance company objected to the cost. When it was reminded of how much money had been invested in the surgery and that the cost of the splints was a fraction of the cost of another surgery, it agreed to pay.

CUTTING THE APRON STRINGS

While the "medical model" approach fosters dependency, the magic of client-centered occupational therapy is in the relationships we forge with our clients. We are equal partners working toward the same goals. Today's clients can be very well-informed about their condition and possible interventions. Computer technology and the Internet provide access to vast amounts of information. Well-informed clients can share information with us to combine it with our specialized knowledge, and together we can design a program that meets the clients' needs and goals.

Encouraging our clients to become independent and self-sufficient extends beyond teaching them how to put on a shirt or go to the bathroom safely. We can teach them how to take good care of their health by encouraging wellness behaviors. We can teach them how to get the most out of their doctor visits. We can help them to understand how to use the health care system responsibly. We can explain how the system works and how they can impact it; for example, teaching clients how to write letters to their representatives in government.

TO BOLDLY GO...

What of the future? Certainly we know that it will be filled with change. With the dawning of a new century and equipped with a client-centered approach, we are free to practice our profession in any environment we choose. While it is unlikely we will totally abandon the traditional practice environments, we have the ability and skill to identify new client groups, to enter into new partnerships, and to enable more people to realize their potential as occupational beings.

Occupational therapists have been practicing in "non-traditional" environments for many years. A 1975 article by Bridle and Bell described their incorporation of community agencies into occupational therapy students' fieldwork experience. At the time, this was a relatively novel idea. Since then, it has become commonplace. At one time, there were no occupational therapists in the school system. Today in the United States, about a quarter of the practicing occupational therapists are employed there. Occupational therapists practice in industry, in independent living programs, in prisons, and in the courts. The difference now is that our future lies in moving away from traditional practice environments in greater numbers.

Cassidy and Kolodner (1999) describe practice in assisted living communities with a focus on prevention strategies and wellness behaviors. Fall prevention, safety awareness, low vision management, adjustment to loss, and environmental modifications define occupational therapy practice in this arena. The Well Elderly Study by Clark and colleagues (1997) is acclaimed as an example of a new arena for occupational therapy. The industrial environment is open to occupational therapists interested in practicing in that sector. As Stricoff (1999) points out, there is a variety of roles we can fill including "consulting, treating, educating, designing, preventing, advocating" (p. 1). Reviewing current practice environments of occupational therapists in the Southeastern United States, Gwin (1999) adds health and wellness programs, senior housing units, welfare-to-work programs, group homes, driver programs, and community accessibility programs to the list. While new practice arenas are exciting, abandonment of our traditional environments is neither practical nor desirable. As responsible health care providers, we must advocate for our clients. We must work to ensure that changes do not deny our clients the health care they need and are entitled to. Susan Scott Lee (1999) makes a compelling case for occupational therapists to be politically active in this regard.

SUMMARY

In this chapter, we demonstrate the relationship between change, costs, cost-restraint measures, policies, politics, and client-centered occupational therapy. As client-centered practitioners, we can encourage responsible use of health care resources, help clients maintain health and wellness, help them to understand the relationship between money and politics, and teach them how to advocate for themselves. The latter may be the best gift we can give them.

ACKNOWLEDGMENTS

We gratefully acknowledge Meg McIntire, OTR/L, CHT, for editorial assistance, Judith Alderton, SROT, DipCOT, for her perspective from the United Kingdom, Alan Bridle, PhD, and Frank Boone, BA, for technical and moral support.

REFERENCES

American Occupational Therapy Association (1999). Health coverage lost as families leave welfare. *OT Week, 31*(21), i-iii.

Benson, H. (1997). *Timeless healing: The power and biology of belief.* New York: Fireside.

Bridle, M.J., & Bell, E.B. (1975). Community placements. *Canadian Journal of Occupational Therapy, 42*(1), 13-15.

Cassidy, J.C., & Kolodner, E.L. (1999). Assisted living 101: Profile of a growth industry. *Gerontology Special Interest Section Quarterly, 22*(June), 1-4.

Clark, F.A., Azen, S.P., Zemke, R., Hackson, J., Carleson, M., Mandel, D., Hay, J., Josepheson, K., Cherry, B., Hessel, C., Palmer, J., & Lipson, L. (1997). Occupational therapy for independent-living older adults: A randomized controlled trial. *Journal of the American Medical Association, 278*(6), 1321-1326.

Fearing, V.G., Clark, J., & Stanton, S. (1998). The client-centered occupational therapy process. In Law, M. (Ed.), *Client-Centered Occupational Therapy* (pp. 67-87). Thorofare, NJ: SLACK Incorporated.

Gwin, C. (1999). AOTA Southeast Regional Program Update. *OT Practice, 4*(6), 57.

Health Canada (1997). *National health expenditures in Canada, 1975-1996.* http://www.hc-sc.gc.ca/datapcb/datahesa/E_expend.htm.

Law, M., Baptiste, S., Carswell, A., McColl, M.A., Polatajko, H., & Pollock, N. (1994). *Canadian Occupational Performance Measure (COPM)* (2nd ed.). Ottawa, Canada: CAOT Publishers.

Novartis Foundation for Gerontological Research (1999). *Putting age on hold: Delaying the diseases of old age.* http://www.healthandage.com/publi/0108020023/page2.htm.

Schaef, A.W. (1996). *Meditations for women who do too much.* New York: HarperCollins.

Scott Lee, S.J. (1999). Lobbying for occupational therapy. *OT Practice, 4*(8), 5-12.

Siebert, C. (1999). Meeting the challenge of new home health care mandates. *OT Practice, 4*(2), 25-29.

Smith, J.S. (1990). *Patenting the sun: Polio and the Salk vaccine.* New York: William Morrow and Co., Inc.

Smyth, C.J., Freyberg, R.H., & McEwen, C. (1985). *History of rheumatology.* Atlanta: Arthritis Foundation.

Statistics Canada. (1997, June). CANSIM database: *Canadian socio-economic information management system.* http://www/datalib./finance/cansim/cansite.htm.

Statistics Canada, Health Canada, Division for Aging and Seniors. (1999). *Canada's Seniors-No. 37: Life expectancy rising and No. 12: Living in institutions.*

Stricoff, R. (1999). The evolution of a solo practitioner's role as a rehabilitation ergonomist within a large corporation. *Work Programs Special Interest Section Quarterly, 13,* 2.

Wythenshawe Hospital Manchester. (1999). *Interesting facts about transplantation.* http://www.nhns.man.ac.uk/NHNSpics.htm.

chapter thirteen

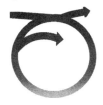

THE USE OF SELF-REFLECTION TO IMPROVE CLIENT-CENTERED PROCESSES

MARLENE STERN, BOT, OT(C), GAYLE RESTALL, MSC, OT (C),
JACQUIE RIPAT, MSC, OT(C)

Reflecting on past events shapes future choices. Take a moment, and think about an event that influenced who you are today. When and where did the event happen? What made the event so significant? Who were the people involved? What were your underlying values and beliefs that affected the way you responded to the event? How did you reflect on the event to make sense of it? As occupational therapists, we are very familiar with the process of reflection. We engage in it daily in our clinical work. We use reflection to critique our clinical work and to problem solve how to do our work better.

In this chapter, the authors again want you to reflect, only this time, the focus will be on client-centered approaches. You will be asked to reflect on what you have learned about client-centered practice, what client-centered practice means to you, your ability to use client-centered approaches, and the milieu in which you use client-centered approaches. This may sound like a lot to think about. It was for us as we began to explore these issues. A great deal was learned about client-centeredness. We discovered that therapists were having difficulty assimilating this approach into practice and that, through discussion and reflection, ways could be found to enhance client-centered approaches. This process eventually led the authors to develop a framework for reflection, called the Client-Centred Process Evaluation (CCPE) (Restall, Stern, & Ripat, 1997), introduced later in this chapter. First, we want you to participate in a reflective journey and think about what you have learned about client-centered practice and some of the challenges you face using client-centered approaches.

CLIENT-CENTERED CONCEPTS

Client-centered, patient-centered, and family-centered are terms that have surfaced in the health care literature as models of service delivery that place the client, patient, or family at the center of the clinical decision-making process. Occupational therapy has embraced the term client-centered practice, and this approach has become a core concept in the occupational therapy process (Canadian Association of Occupational Therapists, 1991, 1994, 1997; Law, 1998). The conceptual basis of client-centered practice has been articulated in these and other documents. Core concepts that have emerged from this literature include developing partnerships with people receiving services, providing clients with informed choices about their health care, facilitating client decision-making, and ensuring that services are accessible and fit into the context of clients' lives. Occupational therapists seem to have accepted client-centered practice as a conceptual model, yet there is evidence to suggest that they have found implementing this approach into daily practice difficult (Brown & Bowen, 1998; Law & Mills, 1998; Neistadt, 1995; Sumsion, 1993).

The authors suggest that the process of reflecting on clinical practice can assist therapists to improve their use of client-centered approaches. We believe that structured reflection consisting of opportunities for therapists to evaluate their own practice, to obtain feedback from their clients, to analyze their practice environments, and to consider alternative strategies for improving practice will assist therapists to discover their own solutions to improving their practice. This chapter will provide a framework for engaging in this reflection.

CHALLENGES IN BEING CLIENT-CENTERED

Implementing client-centered processes can present many challenges even when therapists are committed to it. Understanding the nature of these challenges is fundamental to strategizing ways to enhance client-centered processes. These challenges can be categorized into three broad areas:
1. Personal attributes of the therapist
2. The nature of the relationship between the therapist and client
3. The qualities of the environment in which the therapeutic process takes place

PERSONAL ATTRIBUTES OF THE THERAPIST

Occupational therapists generally strive to behave in a client-centered manner, however, it can be very difficult. A challenge to behaving in a client-centered fashion may be a sincere desire to do what is best for the client. Another may be the therapist's discomfort with client choices. Other sources of uncertainty in behaving in a client-centered manner may be limitations in the existing scientific knowledge base, a limited mastery of its theory, and personal ignorance (Rizzo, 1993). Recognizing the influence of personal attributes, beliefs, and values on the therapy process, and the source of any uncertainty, is critical to using client-centered approaches.

THE RELATIONSHIP BETWEEN THE THERAPIST AND THE CLIENT

The therapeutic process occurs in the context of the relationship between the therapist and the client. This context is shaped by the unique knowledge, skills, expectations, and previous experiences that each brings to the relationship. Some clients may be unable

---

Table 13-1
Components of the Environment

Components	Example of Enablers/Barriers
Physical	Availability of a private treatment room
Social	Models used by other members of the team (e.g., medical model, client-centered practice model)
Cultural	Availability of culturally relevant food items during kitchen assessments
Institutional	Institutional policies about discharge readiness
Socioeconomic	Availability of human resources to provide individual treatment

---

or unwilling to participate in client-centered relationships (Law, Baptiste, & Mills, 1995). With these clients, therapists can be client-centered by using strategies such as graded decision-making and advocacy (Hobson, 1996). With most clients, communication is the key element in articulating and negotiating client-centered relationships. Lack of clear communication makes collaboration with the client in issues such as goal setting difficult (Mew & Fossey, 1996).

THE ENVIRONMENT

Client-centered practice must be considered in the context of the environment in which the therapeutic process takes place. The environment is composed of several components (Law, Cooper, Strong, Stewart, Rigby, & Letts, 1996). The characteristics of these components can work as enablers or barriers to using client-centered approaches (Table 13-1).

Client-centered practice is indeed challenging. Reflection, however, can serve as an important foundation for enhancing client-centered practice, which, in turn, can assist therapists to meet the challenge.

REFLECTION AS A FOUNDATION FOR CLIENT-CENTERED PRACTICE

Reflection is the process of critically evaluating our thinking and acting. Why should therapists reflect on practice? The purpose of reflection is to change behaviors so that professional practice is improved. It is only when therapists reflect on their beliefs, values, behaviors, and relationships with their client, and the environments in which the therapy occurs, will they have the ability to change behavior. Ostermanman and Kottkamp (as cited in Fulmer, 1993) believe that reflective practice is grounded in the belief that all professionals need professional growth opportunities, want to improve and learn, are capable of assuming personal responsibility for learning, and need and want feedback about performance.

Schön (1987) described a way of viewing discrepancies that arise between what therapists would like to do in their practice and what they actually do. Espoused theories are those that therapists articulate and believe guide their practice. Many occupational therapists espouse the principles of client-centered practice. Theories-in-use, however, are more likely to guide much of the professional's behavior. Theories-in-use are culturally based, deeply ingrained, and not easy to articulate. This may explain how many therapists can believe and articulate that client-centered practice is an important, relevant, and effective approach to use in practice (espoused theory), yet have difficulty in implementing this approach in daily practice (theory-in-use).

Consider the many influences on practice. There are many components of clinical reasoning that influence the therapist's decision about the course of action to take in any clinical situation (Schell & Cervero, 1993). The knowledge base that the therapist gained during professional education (Fleming, 1991), the therapist's use of experimentation when his or her current knowledge is insufficient for the given situation (Schön, 1983), and the pragmatic constraints imposed by the work environment (Schell & Cervero, 1993) all serve to influence the therapist's actions. Perhaps more importantly, each therapist brings his or her own beliefs, values, and assumptions about the world into the therapeutic process. These assumptions are often deeply ingrained in the therapist's own sociocultural experience (Hooper, 1997; Schön, 1983).

Reflecting on practice requires commitment and energy. It may take the form of keeping journals, professional portfolios, or having colleagues observe practice or critique videotapes of clinical work. Most therapists engage in some form of reflection during difficult and challenging clinical situations. Commonly, therapists seek feedback from trusted colleagues, problem-solve what they might have done differently to improve the situation, and implement suggestions that they deemed helpful. This process may be helpful for specific situations, but does not necessarily generalize well to other practice areas or address the depth of understanding needed to change theories-in-use that are grounded in often tacit and difficult-to-articulate beliefs and values.

A process of guided reflection that seeks information from a number of sources may offer greater opportunities for therapists to better understand the rationale of their clinical approaches and enhance the use of client-centered practice. The authors have developed the CCPE as a framework to facilitate these opportunities.

OVERVIEW OF THE CCPE

The CCPE encourages therapists to look at their values, beliefs, assumptions, and behaviors, at the therapeutic use of self, at the "professional self," and at their workplace. Continually reflecting upon, clarifying, and improving mental models or internal pictures of the world and how these models shape actions and decisions can assist therapists to become more aware of how they and their environments influence client-centered practice. This discovery can help therapists "see the assumptions and practices that have gone unquestioned for years—and perhaps begin to imagine alternatives" (Senge, Roberts, Rosser, Smith, & Kleiner, 1994, p. 19) to improve client-centered practice.

The CCPE (Appendix C) consists of five sections:
1. Clinician Questionnaire
2. Client Questionnaire
3. Reflection
4. Compilation of Strategies
5. Action Plan

Items for the questionnaires and strategies were generated from an extensive literature review. The review consisted of publications identified earlier in this chapter that were critical to the development of the conceptual model of client-centered practice in occupational therapy; other health care literature that focused on concepts of client-centered, patient-centered, and family-centered care (Chewning, & Sleath, 1996; Coyne, 1996; Gerteis, Edgman-Levitan, Daley, & Delbanco, 1993; King, Rosenbaum, & King, 1996; Rogers, 1957); and literature on transitioning from medical model health care environments to client-centered environments (Engel, 1977; Holden, 1990; Ryden & Rustad, 1985). We also used ideas from therapists generated at interactive workshops at national conferences (Restall & Stern, 1996; Stern & Restall, 1993) and our collective clinical experiences. As the CCPE evolved, we began the process of validating its content through several processes:

- Obtaining feedback through two focus groups consisting of occupational therapists from diverse clinical, academic, and research backgrounds
- Having community lay people critique the client questionnaire for readability and feasibility
- Conducting a pilot test with occupational therapists and clients which included: doing a focus group with the occupational therapist participants after completion of the pilot test; obtaining information from the client participants about the content of the client questionnaire; and doing a follow-up survey of the occupational therapist participants about their changes to practice after using the CCPE

Through a structured process, the CCPE assists the therapist in gathering meaningful information from a variety of sources. This instrument guides therapists to:

- Examine personal client-centered behaviors and the therapeutic relationship with identified clients who participated with the therapist in therapy
- Review the client's perspectives of that relationship
- Explore the discrepancies between what one wants to do and what one does during the therapeutic relationship
- Scan the environment for enablers and constraints to client-centered practice
- Actively plan to make changes to enhance client-centered approaches within and beyond the practice environments

Therapists who choose to use the CCPE are open to introspection and seek to understand the influence of the self on others and the extent to which they are using client-centered approaches. They want this knowledge to determine if there is congruence between what they want to do and what they do. They recognize that insights gained are fundamental for client-centered practice.

The authors invite you to explore your application of the theory of client-centered practice and use the CCPE; completing it will lead to improvements in the use of client-centered approaches and to potentially enhance knowledge about the theory.

CLINICIAN QUESTIONNAIRE

The Clinician Questionnaire is composed of two parts. Part 1, the Therapeutic Process and Relationship, focuses on the direct interaction between you and the client. The items represent behaviors that are conceptually congruent with client-centered practice and are structured around the therapeutic process. Fearing, Law, and Clark (1997) have described seven stages of the Occupational Performance Process Model. Each stage of the therapeutic process offers unique and important opportunities for implementing client-centered approaches. The clinician questionnaire was developed using stages of the therapeutic process as a basis for describing various client-centered activities to assist you in an examination of your client-centered behaviors in a systematic and structured manner. A visual analogue scale is used for you to record your responses.

Part 2, the Environmental Scan, is an examination of the work environment. Law (1991) describes the environment as "those contexts and situations which occur outside the individual and elicits response from them" (p. 175). The Environmental Scan examines the physical, social, cultural, institutional, and socioeconomic components of the work environment. You are to consider the organization that employs you to provide clinical services, respond to 24 statements with either a true or false, and to decide whether the answer to each statement enables, is a barrier to, or is not relevant to being client-centered.

CLIENT QUESTIONNAIRE

You begin by requesting that a client participate and complete the client questionnaire. The client may be the actual consumer of the services provided, a primary caregiver of the identified consumer, or another individual or group who has the authority to influence and direct therapy (e.g., a third party payer). The client must have sufficient comprehension of the English language and an understanding of the purpose of the questionnaire and must agree to return it once completed to you. Client participants should have completed or be nearing the end of the therapeutic process with you to allow examination of the entire therapeutic process.

The Client Questionnaire consists of two parts: the Therapeutic Process and Relationship and the Environmental Scan. Part 1 asks the client to comment on his or her perception of the relationship with you based on a number of criteria, using a 4-point Likert scale. The items in the questionnaire focus on respect, communication between you and your client, shared responsibility for therapy, and involvement of the people important in your client's life. Part 2 asks the client for his or her perception about the environment in which therapy occurred.

REFLECTION

The reflection component is the heart of the framework. Through guided reflection, you are encouraged to examine the responses to the Client and Clinician Questionnaires. A Reflection Summary Form is provided to record the responses. The intent is not to calculate aggregate scores but rather to facilitate your reflection on client-centered processes. On the Summary Form, you identify the items from the Client Questionnaire, Part 1, the Therapeutic Process and Relationship, that the client rated negatively. You also identify the items on the Clinician Questionnaire, Part 1, the Therapeutic Process and Relationship, that you rated poorly. Next, characteristics of the environment that you or the client identified as being either enablers or barriers are documented. At this point, you will have a summary of the responses from the questionnaires. It is important to remember that any given response should not be considered a grade of client-centered practice. Instead, you are encouraged to consider each item and reflect on whether, in the specific context of your therapeutic involvement with the client, you were being client-centered.

Occupational therapists who attended the focus groups and provided feedback about the CCPE spoke of the benefits of guided reflection. The opportunity to analyze one's own behaviors and work environment and to receive client feedback was a powerful and meaningful experience for therapist participants. Participants told us:

> *It made me think...did I tell them what I recommended, did I ask them to agree with what we were doing, did I enter into a situation where that was implicit or did I say, "Well this is what I think, what do you think?"*

> *I think for me it is easy to say, yes, I am trying to work in a client-centered manner. But having these questions to reflect on guided me as to where I am client-centered and where I'm not. It also helped as to how I could change the course of how I am doing things with some clients, recognizing that it would work better with some clients than with others. But even with the ones where it doesn't work all that well, there are some specific questions that helped steer me in a more client-centered manner. So I think that it's really good.*

> *I really like the Environmental Scan because I don't know how to answer it. I think it makes me realize where I can ask questions and identify better the environment that I am working in.*

Through reflection, the framework makes explicit the approaches and systems that can influence therapist interactions and behaviors with the client, which are both significant contributors to client-centered practice.

Meaningful reflection, however, requires that you take the time to make sense of and be open to the responses. Recall that your analysis of the responses will be influenced by a number of factors including your own and your workplace's knowledge of values, beliefs, and assumptions about client-centered practice and the therapeutic relationship with your client. New information, experiences, and reflection will cause these factors to shift over time. Although you may have the urge to say "yes, but..." and attach qualifying information to the responses, we encourage you to suspend assumptions and spend the time reflecting about what the information can teach you and what actions you want to pursue. Try not to rush through this stage, as it is here that you will bring the information, your thoughts, and ideas together and develop a plan to guide future practice. If you don't spend enough time reflecting, you might draw premature conclusions and develop irrelevant action plans.

COMPILATION OF STRATEGIES

The next step is to review the Compilation of Strategies. Fifty strategies are organized into six categories. These strategies are offered as ideas for you to consider when developing the final stage of the process, the Action Plan. The strategies are not linear; you can start at any part of the circle. However, you will find that they progress from strategies that focus on personal work through to collaborative advocacy strategies in the political arena. A definition of each category and a few examples follow.

- **Personal reflection is the process of cognitively and effectively exploring clinical experience to gain greater insight into client-centered practice.** Using the CCPE is one way for you to reflect on your practice. You may develop an action plan that includes the use of the CCPE on multiple occasions and with multiple clients. Other methods of personal reflection can also be part of the action plan. These methods may include keeping a reflective professional journal or seeking feedback from a trusted professional colleague. Enhancing your perspective of the illness experience is another approach. Clients have recommended that service providers be educated in a manner that gives service providers a "gut level" understanding of illness and its effect on the individual (Corring & Cook, 1999).
- **Facilitating client-centered processes is the therapist's active and conscious facilitation of client-centered interactions between the therapist and client.** For example, after completing the CCPE, you may discover that your client felt that you did not focus on issues that he or she thought important. You may decide to use the Canadian Occupational Performance Measure (COPM) (Law, Baptiste, Carswell, McColl, Polatajko, & Pollock, 1994) in future assessments. You may then be attentive to ensuring that the issues of high priority to your client are a primary focus of therapy.
- **Developing client-centered practice settings is the process of developing a practice environment conducive to client-centered approaches.** This strategy involves making changes within the practice environment. An example is to make changes to job descriptions so that facilitation of client involvement in therapy decisions is a requirement. Another example is to include former clients in the development of program evaluation processes.
- **Community organization is the process of organizing people around client-centered practice issues or problems that are larger than any one individual's immediate concerns** (Registered Nurses Association of British Columbia [RNABC], 1992). This group of strategies involves the public in having influence over health delivery issues. It can include conducting community needs assessments and the establishment of client advisory committees to facilitate client input in the delivery of health services.
- **Coalition advocacy is the bringing together of diverse groups temporarily to advocate for policies and reforms that support client-centered practice** (RNABC, 1992). This group of strategies focuses on influencing policy makers to create environments that are more conducive to client-centered practice. It presumes that advocacy by clinicians from a variety of professions, together with clients, can be more successful than groups lobbying on behalf of homogeneous groups.

- **Political action is similar to coalition advocacy, however, it focuses on social change and networking, particularly to elected politicians** (RNABC, 1992). Imagine the strength of a united voice of diverse groups collectively lobbying politicians to promote or entrench client-centered care approaches as central to health care services. As an example, consider the successful efforts realized by both homogeneous and diverse groups working together to obtain legislative reforms such as improved accessibility for the disabled, smoking laws, and stronger penalties to impaired drivers.

ACTION PLAN

The final step of the CCPE is the development of an Action Plan. This is where you translate your reflections about the therapeutic process, the environment, and the strategies into action steps. You commit to a plan that outlines the ways in which you will improve your client-centered approaches.

The therapists who participated in the pilot study received follow-up surveys that asked questions about changes made to their client-centered approaches since completing the CCPE. Comments related to implementing the identified action plans included:

> *Some of my action plans were immediate (e.g., providing clients with informed options), and this has been instituted with new clients. My other action plan regarding team philosophy (specifically educating physicians regarding client-centeredness) is underway. This was a goal I had prior to the CCPE, but likely undertaking the CCPE helped to reiterate the importance of this client-centered approach.*

> *Started using the COPM. Also have become more aware of involving the client (even more).*

APPLICATION TO PRACTICE

The structured reflection (i.e., that is the core of the CCPE) lends itself to a wide variety of applications. Novice and expert therapists may find the CCPE assists in an examination of their own practice and practice environment. Therapists at the focus groups spoke about using the CCPE to examine a particularly challenging clinical situation in greater detail. By considering the barriers and enablers to client-centered practice in the therapeutic relationship and within the environment, the therapist can take a clear and objective look at the situation. By using guided reflection, he or she may be able to identify a particular situation that is preventing the therapeutic relationship from moving forward. One therapist at a focus group commented:

> *I think (it) might be useful when you get stuck—because it's a way of you taking a look at what you're doing and getting your client's feedback and putting it together.*

Therapists involved in the focus groups identified that the CCPE would be useful for students on fieldwork placements. Students will have been introduced to the theoretical basis of client-centered practice during their education but may be unclear how to implement the concepts in a clinical situation. Using the CCPE may assist in their professional growth and development in the use of client-centered approaches.

> *I think it would be a great thing to do with students [who] come through your agency on placement...[it] teaches the student to look at each and every clinical setting [he or she goes] into this way.*

The CCPE may be used to educate team members on client-centered practice in a manner that helps to simplify a potentially complex concept. Clinical teams can use the CCPE with a variety of clients to compile feedback that can be used as an indicator of the program's ability to operate from a client-centered perspective. Health care professionals indoctrinated in the medical model may have difficulty in shifting their approach to a client-centered one. They may struggle with putting client-centered theory into practice and may use the CCPE as a method of determining ways that the program can implement the concepts. A participant in a focus group described the challenge this way:

> *I would use this tool to get (others) interested about the topic. I think client-centered is one of those topics in occupational therapy that a lot of people don't know...It is so complicated—it exhausts people I think.*

The CCPE could be used as a communication tool with the team to bring forward client thoughts and feelings. It could be used to assist the team to understand the client's perspective through direct client feedback. If used in this manner, the client may be asked to complete the Client Questionnaire considering the team as a whole. One focus group participant described this use of the CCPE as follows:

> *...Bringing that information...to the team setting so that...other people [are made] more aware perhaps where a client's not feeling that things are being very client-centered...*

Occupational therapy graduate students and researchers may choose to use the CCPE as a tool to further explore and define the concepts of client-centered practice. The tool lends itself to examining both therapist-client relationship and program conditions that either support or prevent the use of client-centered approaches. Senge et al. (1994) suggest that the cycle of developing theories and creating and applying practical methods and tools based on the theories leads to new insights that improve the theory. Insights gained from using the CCPE have the potential to enhance the theory of client-centered practice.

The primary intent of the CCPE is that it be used as a tool for reflection for therapists and students involved in direct client intervention. Supervisors and educators can encourage the use of the CCPE to evaluate performance and develop client-centered expertise in staff and students. Accumulation of knowledge of client-centered practice through the use of the CCPE as a research tool can augment the reflection process by providing greater clarity about the meaning of client-centered practice. Thus, the CCPE has a broad range of applications for therapists, students, managers, educators, and researchers.

CASE EXAMPLE

To further illustrate the potential application to practice, consider the following case example. Jason is a 23-year-old truck driver who had an acquired brain injury as a result of a work-related accident. He was an inpatient on a brain injury unit in a rehabilitation hospital. As a result of the injury, Jason had significant short-term memory loss, impaired insight, and decreased initiation. During multidisciplinary team rounds, several team members expressed concerns that Jason had not been attending therapy sessions. He was often spotted in the cafeteria with his girlfriend instead of attending his appointments. The physician informed the team that he would insist that Jason begin to attend therapy. Despite this plan, Jason's attendance at therapy remained inconsistent. Tracy, his occupational therapist, was concerned that Jason would not meet the goals that had been set for him by the team in the initial assessment conference prior to his discharge.

Tracy wondered why Jason did not seem committed to participating in therapy and achieving the goals they had set. She decided to complete the CCPE to identify potential areas in which she was not practicing in a client-centered manner and to obtain Jason's feedback on her behavior.

After completing the CCPE, Tracy identified several areas of concern. On the Client Questionnaire, Jason identified that he did not feel Tracy focused on the issues that he felt were important and that she did not always respect the choices he made. In the comment section, he stated that he did not feel he could live up to her expectations. In addition, Jason indicated that he did not feel that she was open, honest, and timely with information and commented that he felt the team was "hiding" things from him. Jason indicated that he felt uncomfortable in the environment in which he received therapy because he did not like to talk about personal issues in the large therapy room that lacked privacy.

Tracy completed the Clinician Questionnaire and also identified some areas in which she had not acted in a client-centered manner throughout the therapeutic process. She realized that she did not provide Jason with much information about the range of services that she could offer him and had not explicitly talked to him about the expectations that he be an active participant in the therapeutic process. Through the Environmental Scan, Tracy recognized that members of the team had differing philosophies about the use of client-centered approaches. Some team members did not believe that clients should be active decision-makers in their treatment. She also recognized that the team did not often discuss these differences in philosophy or the potential benefit of using a more client-centered approach. After a review of her job description, Tracy noted that there was no reference to collaborating with clients as an expectation. However, Tracy was aware that her

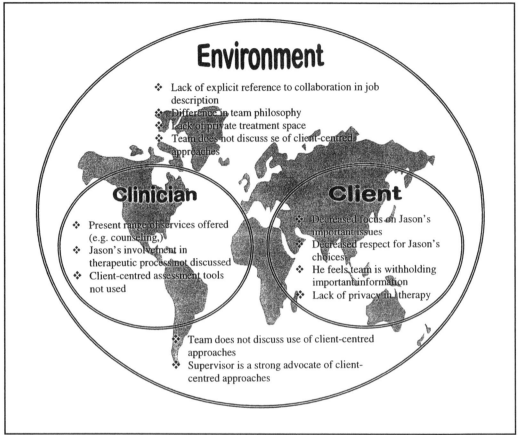

Figure 13-1. Sample Reflection Summary Form.

supervisor was a strong advocate of client-centered approaches and could be a potential source of support to implementing these approaches within the team.

Tracy reflected on her personal approach, her therapeutic relationship with Jason and her other clients, and the environment in which she practiced. She was aware that she valued the concepts of client-centered practice and wanted to make changes to how she implemented these with her clients. After summarizing the results of the CCPE in the Reflection Summary Form (Figure 13-1) and reviewing the Compilation of Strategies, Tracy developed the following Action Plan (Table 13-2).

Tracy administered the COPM as she had outlined in her Action Plan, and Jason identified five occupational performance goals that were important for him to work on while at the rehabilitation center. She located a private room where they could meet for therapy sessions. Subsequently, Jason appeared to become more invested in his therapy as indicated by his improved attendance at sessions and involvement in decision-making. He initiated a discharge team conference and identified the primary issues that he felt needed discussion. Tracy continued to work through her Action Plan after Jason's discharge and facilitated an inservice and discussion with her team on client-centered strategies. She continued to work on developing her client-centered approaches and decided to use the CCPE to receive feedback and to reflect on her progress on an annual basis.

Table 13-2
Sample Action Plan

Priority	Plan	Timeline
1	Administer COPM	End of next week
4	Educate team on client-centered theory	End of month
5	Ask supervisor to sit in on a therapy session and provide feedback on approaches	Next referral
3	Volunteer to sit on Rehabilitation Center committee for family-centered care	Immediately
2	Speak to team leader about setting up a private therapy space	Immediately

SUMMARY

Becoming a client-centered therapist requires reflection and the commitment to translate insights gained into practice. The authors developed the CCPE to assist in this reflective journey. We hope that you will find it useful. We will continue to develop the CCPE as a reliable and valid tool. The authors invite your feedback and comments on its content and application to assist with our journey. Further information and instructions on using the CCPE are also available from the authors. They can be reached through SLACK Incorporated, 6900 Grove Road, Thorofare, NJ 08086; website: www.slackbooks.com.

REFERENCES

Brown, C., & Bowen, R. (1998). Including consumer and environment in occupational therapy treatment planning. *Occupational Therapy Journal of Research, 18,* 44-62.

Canadian Association of Occupational Therapists (1991). *Occupational therapy guidelines for client-centred practice.* Toronto, Ontario, Canada: CAOT Publications ACE.

Canadian Association of Occupational Therapists (1994). *Occupational therapy guidelines for client-centred mental health practice.* Toronto, Ontario, Canada: CAOT Publications ACE.

Canadian Association of Occupational Therapists (1997). *Enabling occupation: An occupational therapy perspective.* Ottawa, Ontario, Canada: CAOT Publications ACE.

Chewning, B., & Sleath, B. (1996). Medication decision-making and management: A client-centred model. *Social Science and Medicine, 42,* 389-398.

Corring, D., & Cook, J. (1999). Client-centred care means that I am a valued human being. *Canadian Journal of Occupational Therapy, 66,* 71-82.

Coyne, I. (1996). Parent participation: A concept analysis. *Journal of Advanced Nursing, 23,* 733-740.

Engel, G. (1977). The need for a new medical model: A challenge for biomedicine. *Science, 196,* 129-136.

Fearing, V.G., Law, M., & Clark, J. (1997). An occupational performance process model: Fostering client and therapist alliances. *Canadian Journal of Occupational Therapy, 64,* 7-15.

Fleming, M. (1991). The therapist with the three-track mind. *American Journal of Occupational Therapy, 45,* 1007-1014.

Fulmer, C. (1993). Developing a reflective practice of professional development. *School Business Affairs, September,* 23-26.

Gerteis, M., Edgman-Levitan, S., Daley, J., & Delbanco, T. (Eds.). (1993). *Through the patient's eyes: Understanding and promoting patient-centred care*. San Francisco: Jossey-Bass.

Hobson, S. (1996). Being client-centered when the client is cognitively impaired. *Canadian Journal of Occupational Therapy, 63*, 133-137.

Holden, R. (1990). Models, muddles and medicine. *International Journal of Nursing Studies, 27*, 223-234.

Hooper, B. (1997). The relationship between pretheoretical assumptions and clinical reasoning. *American Journal of Occupational Therapy, 51*, 328-338.

King, S., Rosenbaum, P., & King, G. (1996). Parent's perceptions of caregiving: Development and validation of a measure of processes. *Developmental Medicine and Child Neurology, 38*, 757-772.

Law, M. (1991). The environment: A focus for occupational therapy. *Canadian Journal of Occupational Therapy, 58*(4), 171-179.

Law, M. (Ed.). (1998). *Client-centered occupational therapy*. Thorofare, NJ: SLACK Incorporated.

Law, M., Baptiste, S., Carswell, A., McColl, M.A., Polatajko, H., & Pollock, N. (1994). *Canadian Occupational Performance Measure manual (COPM)* (2nd ed.). Toronto, Ontario, Canada: CAOT Publications ACE.

Law, M., Baptiste, S., & Mills, J. (1995). Client-centred practice: What does it mean and does it make a difference? *Canadian Journal of Occupational Therapy, 62*, 250-257.

Law, M., Cooper, B., Strong, S., Stewart, D., Rigby, P., & Letts, L. (1996). The Person-Environment-Occupation model: A transactive approach to occupational performance. *Canadian Journal of Occupational Therapy, 63*, 9-23.

Law, M., & Mills, J. (1998). Client-centred occupational therapy. In M. Law (Ed.), *Client-Centered Occupational Therapy* (pp. 2-18). Thorofare, NJ: SLACK Incorporated.

Mew, M., & Fossey, E. (1996). Client-centred aspects of clinical reasoning during an initial assessment using the Canadian Occupational Performance Measure. *Australian Occupational Therapy Journal, 43*, 155-166.

Neistadt, M. (1995). Methods of assessing clients' priorities: A survey of adult physical dysfunction settings. *American Journal of Occupational Therapy, 49*, 428-436.

Registered Nurses Association of British Columbia (1992). *Determinants of health: Empowering strategies for nursing practice*. Vancouver, British Columbia, Canada: Author.

Restall, G., & Stern, M. (1996, April). *Being client-centred in a medical model environment*. Short course presented at the annual meeting of the American Occupational Therapy Association, Chicago.

Restall, G., Stern, M., & Ripat, J. (1997). *The client-centred process evaluation*. Unpublished document.

Rizzo, J. (1993). Physician uncertainty and the art of persuasion. *Social Science and Medicine, 37*, 1451-1459.

Rogers, C. (1957). The necessary and sufficient conditions of therapeutic personality change. *Journal of Consulting Psychology, 21*(2), 95-103.

Ryden, M., & Rustad, R. (1985). Wellness model replaces medical model. *Journal of Long-Term Care Administration, 13*, 115-119.

Schell, B., & Cervero, R. (1993). Clinical reasoning in occupational therapy: An integrative review. *American Journal of Occupational Therapy, 47*, 605-610.

Schön, D. (1983). *The reflective practitioner: How professionals think in action*. New York: Basic Books.

Schön, D. (1987). *Educating the reflective practitioner*. San Francisco: Jossey-Bass.

Senge, P., Roberts, C., Rosser, B., Smith, B.J., & Kleiner, A. (1994). *The fifth discipline fieldbook*. New York: Doubleday.

Stern, M., & Restall, G. (1993, June). *Client-centred practice and the medical model*. Paper presented at the annual meeting of the Canadian Association of Occupational Therapists. Regina, Saskatchewan, Canada.

Sumsion, T. (1993). Client-centred practice: The true impact. *Canadian Journal of Occupational Therapy, 60*, 6-8.

appendix a

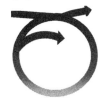

GUIDELINES FOR CLIENT-CENTERED PROGRAMS

1.0 RATIONALE

The purpose for program rationale, generally on a page or less, is to identify:

- Client unmet needs and expectations related to occupational performance
- Potential outcomes and benefits to clients and others
- Currently available resources/programs
- Numbers of people with occupational performance needs and their locations
- Scientific evidence that supports this type of program

2.0 OUTCOME

2.1 EXPECTED OUTCOME

An expected outcome is a best estimate of what will result at some future time from activity or process (or lack of it). Expected outcomes meet the following criteria:

- **Client-centered.** Expected outcomes are stated from the client's point of view
- **Occupational performance.** Expected outcomes involve occupational performance that is valued by the client
- **Behavioral.** Expected outcomes are stated in behavioral terms so that it will be possible to recognize when the outcome has been achieved
- **Time limited.** Expected outcomes have meaning within the context of a time frame

2.2 OBJECTIVES

Objectives are key client behaviors that should be attained to achieve the expected client outcome. Objectives meet the following criteria:

- Realistic
- Understandable
- Measurable
- Behavioral
- Achievable

2.3 OUTCOME MEASURE(S)

To evaluate program outcome:
- Compare expected outcome with actual outcome
- Evaluate client satisfaction with performance (e.g., COPM)
- If program standards have been set, compare standard with actual outcome

3.0 PROCESS
(THIS SECTION IS A CLINICAL PROTOCOL)

Referral

State:
- Eligibility criteria for the program
- Number of clients who can be in the program at any one time
- How referrals are received
- Forms used and procedure regarding completion
- Documentation procedure following receipt of the referral

3.1 SCREENING:
NAME, VALIDATE, AND PRIORITIZE OPIs

State:
- Typical OPIs identified during screening
- Method used to gather information about OPIs
- Method used to validate these issues and determine order of importance to the client
- Action taken if there are no OPIs of importance to the client

3.2 SELECT THEORETICAL APPROACHES

State:
- Identify theoretical approaches to be used (e.g., biomechanical, environmental). This influences the assessment tools selected as well as the intervention approach

3.3 IDENTIFY OCCUPATIONAL PERFORMANCE
COMPONENTS AND ENVIRONMENTAL CONDITIONS

State:
- Assessments that may be used to understand the reasons for OPIs related to this program. Identify components contributing to the OPIs
- Method of referral to other disciplines for necessary assessment
- Procedure regarding documentation of assessment information

3.4 IDENTIFY STRENGTHS AND RESOURCES

State:
- Client resources
- Therapist resources
- Social and environmental resources that are available

3.5 NEGOTIATE TARGETED OUTCOMES AND DEVELOP ACTION PLANS

State:
- How individual outcomes can be met through program process
- Method used for negotiating with clients
- Actions that must occur to achieve objectives and outcomes
- Staff and client responsibility for action

3.6 IMPLEMENT PLANS THROUGH OCCUPATION

State:
- Actions planned to address each objective identified
- Factors considered in implementing the program
- Method for determining whether planned actions have meaning to the clients
- Procedure regarding frequency of reassessment
- Procedure regarding team/family communication
- Procedure regarding frequency of documentation

3.7 EVALUATE OCCUPATIONAL PERFORMANCE OUTCOMES

State:
- How individual client outcomes will be evaluated. This may be different than the method used to evaluate program outcome (see 2.3)
- Procedure used when outcomes have not been met
- Procedure used when outcomes have been met

3.8 FOLLOW-UP

State:
- Procedure regarding provision of follow-up
- Mechanism for coordinating further services, if necessary

3.9 PROCESS MEASUREMENT

State:
- Method for reviewing adherence to program process as outlined in Section 3

4.0 STRUCTURE

4.1 PERSONNEL

State:
- Competencies required of personnel
- Responsibilities of each person
- Reporting structure for the personnel in this program

4.2 SPACE

State:
- Program location
- Accessibility facts
- Schedule for use of space

4.3 BUDGET

State:
- Operating costs
- Capital costs
- Revenue to be expected

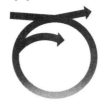

OCCUPATIONAL THERAPY STANDARDS: CLINICAL RECORDS

A health record is the cumulative health diary of one client. Information entered into that record remains there to be read by the client and all other people who have access to the record. It is a serious responsibility to document on a client's health record in such a way that the information has meaning to the client and to others.

STANDARD 1

Occupational therapists will meet VHHSC corporate clinical record documentation standards.

STANDARD 2

Occupational therapists will concisely document the client-centered occupational therapy problem-solving process.

- Record actual or potential **OPIs** that are important to the client. This is often recorded on a problem list. This information is profession specific.
- Record assessment data that identify **components and conditions that contribute to identified OPIs**. This is generally recorded in the data base section of the health record.
- Record client **strengths and resources** that may be woven into the intervention plan. This is usually recorded in the data base section as part of assessment information.
- Record **targeted outcomes** identified in collaboration with the client. This outcome may be, for example, "Return home by September 15, 2001." It includes a projected timeline as well as a vision for the future. Make an action plan that identifies **who** will do **what**. The targeted outcome is often recorded on the problem list while the action plan is recorded in progress notes.
- Record action plan and the results of the implementation of the action plan. This includes the **when, where**, and **how**. This information is generally recorded in the progress notes.
- Record **resolution of OPIs** and/or components. This is an effective outcome measure. It is usually recorded on the problem list.

appendix c

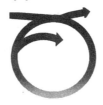

CLIENT-CENTRED PROCESS EVALUATION

SECTION 1 OF 5:
CLINICIAN QUESTIONNAIRE

PART 1, THERAPEUTIC PROCESS AND RELATIONSHIP

Please circle the answer that reflects your thoughts about your experiences providing services to _____. Please try to answer all questions. If any questions do not apply to your experiences, please leave them blank.

1. Did you provide your client with information about the clinical services that you had to offer?

1	2	3	4	5
Definitely				Definitely not

2. Did you discuss with your client your expectations for his or her involvement in the therapeutic process?

1	2	3	4	5
Definitely				Definitely not

3. Did you involve your client in identifying the problems that he or she wanted to address in therapy?

1	2	3	4	5
Definitely				Definitely not

4. Did you seek your client's opinion about which problems were most meaningful to him or her?

1	2	3	4	5
Definitely				Definitely not

5. Did you discuss with your client the potential risk of NOT addressing a particular problem in therapy?

1   2   3   4   5
Definitely   Definitely not

6. Did you assist your client in identifying his or her strengths that could be used to achieve the goals?

1   2   3   4   5
Definitely   Definitely not

7. Did you involve your client in setting therapy goals?

1   2   3   4   5
Definitely   Definitely not

8. Did you assist your client in identifying his or her resources that could be used to achieve his or her goals?

1   2   3   4   5
Definitely   Definitely not

9. Did you give your client information about the advantages and disadvantages of each intervention that you recommended for achieving the goals?

1   2   3   4   5
Definitely   Definitely not

10. Did you negotiate a course of action for reaching therapy goals with your client?

1   2   3   4   5
Definitely   Definitely not

11. Did you involve your client in modifying the course of action during the therapeutic process?

1   2   3   4   5
Definitely   Definitely not

12. Did you and your client agree that the identified therapy goals had been achieved?

1   2   3   4   5
Definitely   Definitely not

13. Did you and your client agree that he or she was ready for discharge from therapy?

1	2	3	4	5
Definitely				Definitely not

14. Did you provide information to your client about how to access other services he or she needed?

1	2	3	4	5
Definitely				Definitely not

15. Did you seek your client's opinion about whether therapy was effective?

1	2	3	4	5
Definitely				Definitely not

16. Did you involve your client in decisions about future contact or follow-up?

1	2	3	4	5
Definitely				Definitely not

17. Do you feel your client felt comfortable disagreeing with you during the therapeutic process?

1	2	3	4	5
Definitely				Definitely not

18. Was it important to you to involve your client in making decisions about his or her therapy?

1	2	3	4	5
Definitely				Definitely not

19. What supported or prevented your ability to be client-centred in the therapeutic process with your client?

20. Comments:

PART 2, ENVIRONMENTAL SCAN

In completing the Environmental Scan survey, you are asked to consider the organization that directly employs you to provide clinical services. Specifically, reflect on the organizational structures, systems, and processes that influence the provision of services to clients. Please indicate whether each of the following statements is true or false for your work environment and whether each component in your work environment is a barrier, a support, or not relevant to your ability to be client-centred with this client. Circle your responses.

Component	True (T) or False (F)	Barrier (B) or Support (S) or Not Relevant (N)
1. Mission Statement The mission statement that guides your practice refers to providing services in collaboration with clients.	T F	B S N
2. Your Supervisor's Philosophy Your supervisor demonstrates a commitment to the use of client-centred approaches.	T F	B S N
3. Management Philosophy The management of the organization demonstrates a commitment to the use of client-centred approaches.	T F	B S N
4. Job Descriptions Your job description explicitly lists collaboration with clients as a major responsibility.	T F	B S N
5. Staff Orientation Staff receive an orientation to the organization's expectations for client-centred practice.	T F	B S N
6. Student Orientation Students receive an orientation to the organization's expectations for client-centred practice.	T F	B S N

Restall, G., Stern M., & Ripat, J. *The Client-Centred Process Evaluation.* © 1997.

7. Performance Appraisals   T F   B S N
Your performance appraisal includes
evaluations of your use of
client-centred approaches.

8. Student Appraisals   T F   B S N
Appraisals of students include evaluations
of the use of client-centred approaches.

9. Direct Access   T F   B S N
Clients have direct access to your services
without referral from another professional
(e.g., physician, nurse, etc.).

10. Choice of Health Care Providers   T F   B S N
Clients are able to choose the clinician from
whom they receive service in your organization.

11. Accessibility   T F   B S N
Clinical services are in a location that
is easily accessible to clients.

12. Clinical Setting   T F   B S N
Clinical services are provided in the setting
that can optimally address the client's
therapeutic needs and desires.

13. Availability of Physical Resources   T F   B S N
Supply and equipment resources are
available to provide clients with options.

14. Time Frame   T F   B S N
There is sufficient time to collaborate with
clients throughout the therapeutic process.

15. Organizational Decision-Making   T F   B S N
Clinicians are empowered to participate in
decisions that affect them within the
organization.

16. Cultural Sensitivity   T F   B S N
There is an explicit commitment to providing
services that respect and accommodate
the cultural background of clients.

17. Client Assessment Tools   T F   B S N
A client assessment tool is available for your
use within your organization that is based on
the concepts of client-centred practice.

18. Outcome Measures   T F   B S N
An outcome measure is available for your use
within your organization that includes items
related to the clients' perspective on their
therapeutic outcome.

19. Availability of Human Resources T F   B S N
Sufficient staff are available to provide clients
with opportunities to work on their established
goals.

20. Team Philosophy   T F   B S N
The client's health care providers all support
the use of client-centred approaches.

21. Team Discussions   T F   B S N
There are opportunities for clinicians to
discuss issues and conflicts related to being
client-centred.

22. Community Involvement   T F   B S N
The organization implements strategies
identified by the community to
address health needs.

23. Data Collection Systems   T F   B S N
Your workload recording system has
data entry fields to record statistics when
your client is an individual, a family, an agency,
and a community.

24. Health Care Funding   T F   B S N

Clients and clinicians are able to
collaboratively decide the length and
nature of intervention without limitations
set by funding sources
(e.g., public or private insurance agencies).

SECTION 2 OF 5
CLIENT QUESTIONNAIRE

PART 1, THERAPEUTIC PROCESS AND RELATIONSHIP

Read each statement. Circle the response that best reflects your feelings. Feel free to make comments in the space below each statement.

1. Your therapist treated you as a unique individual.

Not at all   A little   Quite a bit   A lot

Comments:

2. Your therapist tried to understand how your problem affected your day-to-day life.

Not at all   A little   Quite a bit   A lot

Comments:

3. Your therapist focused on the issues that you felt were important.

Not at all   A little   Quite a bit   A lot

Comments:

4. You had enough control over what happened during your therapy.

Not at all   A little   Quite a bit   A lot

Comments:

5. Your therapist respected the choices you made.

Not at all   A little   Quite a bit   A lot

Comments:

6. Your therapist helped you discover your potential.

Not at all   A little   Quite a bit   A lot

Comments:

7. **Your therapist encouraged you to share responsibility for what happened during your therapy.**

Not at all   A little   Quite a bit   A lot
Comments:

8. **Your therapist was open, honest, and timely with information.**

Not at all   A little   Quite a bit   A lot
Comments:

9. **The important people in your life were given the opportunity to be involved in your therapy.**

Not at all   A little   Quite a bit   A lot
Comments:

10. **You trusted your therapist.**

Not at all   A little   Quite a bit   A lot
Comments:

PART 2, ENVIRONMENTAL SCAN

1. **You felt comfortable in the place in which you received therapy.**

Not at all   A little   Quite a bit   A lot
Comments:

2. **Therapy occurred in the most appropriate place (e.g., the ward, the therapy department, or your home).**

Strongly agree   Agree   Disagree   Strongly disagree
Comments:

3. **There was enough communication between all of the people involved in your care.**

Strongly agree   Agree   Disagree   Strongly disagree
Comments:

Thank you for taking the time to complete this survey!

Restall, G., Stern M., & Ripat, J. *The Client-Centred Process Evaluation.* © 1997.

SECTION 3 OF 5
REFLECTION SUMMARY FORM

Use this form to collect your responses, thoughts, and ideas. You will use this information to develop your action plan.

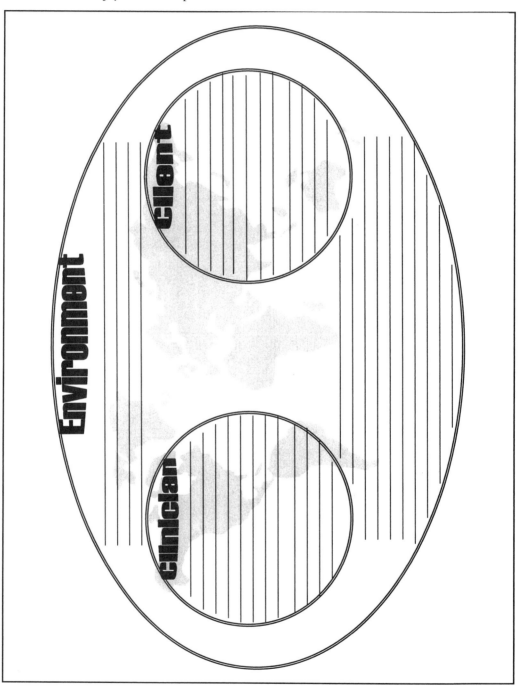

SECTION 4 OF 5
COMPILATION OF STRATEGIES

Personal Reflection (cognitively and effectively exploring clinical experiences in order to gain greater insight into client-centred practice).

- Read the literature on client-centred practice
- Network with others who are interested in client-centred practice
- Participate in professional development opportunities related to client-centred practice
- Ask colleagues to observe and critique your practice
- Observe colleagues' practice
- Tell stories about the use of client-centred practice
- Become involved with professional organizations
- Identify the real client
- Clarify and understand your own values
- Develop your understanding about where and with whom you have influence
- Develop diversity within your practice
- Reflect on whether your philosophy of client-centred practice is congruent with your employer's use of client-centred language
- Develop your own self-esteem

Client-Centred Processes (facilitating client-centred interactions between clinician and client).

- Review assessments and documentation to determine if they are congruent with client-centred practice
- Use client-centred outcome measures (e.g., COPM)
- Conduct outcome studies that investigate the relationship between client-centred practice and therapy outcome, cost-effectiveness, efficiency, etc.
- Educate clients about client-centred approaches
- Facilitate clients' reflection on their own values
- Teach client advocacy skills
- Coach and encourage clients to question health care providers
- Provide interventions in an environment that is meaningful to the client

Practice Settings (developing a practice environment conducive to client-centred approaches).

- Review mission statements, job descriptions, performance appraisals, and policies; make or advocate for changes that would support client-centred processes
- Incorporate client perspectives into program planning and evaluation
- Report on use and outcomes of client-centred approaches
- Model client-centred practice to colleagues in the practice setting
- Organize colleagues around client-centred issues or problems with the goal of improving service quality

---

- Talk about client-centred practice and its impact within practice settings
- Review approaches to client-centred practice used by other organizations
- Establish support networks for client-centred practice within the practice environment
- Learn from strategies used by others

Community Organizations (organizing people around client-centered practice issues or problems that are larger than your immediate concerns).
- Knock on doors
- Write media releases
- Engage in critical dialogue about professional practices
- Draft and circulate policies and position statements that support client-centered practice
- Conduct community needs assessments
- Serve as a resource to community/self-help groups
- Engage in community development activities
- Form client advisory committees

Coalition Advocacy (bringing together diverse groups temporarily to advocate for policies and reforms that support client-centered practice).
- Collaborate with other health care providers and provincial associations around client-centered practice issues
- Advocate for client-centered friendly funding methods (e.g., individualized brokerage system)
- Speak publicly about client-centered issues
- Contact the media for the purpose of communicating the position on a client-centered practice issue
- Network with other groups, organizations, and government bodies
- Lend support to community and self-help groups who support client-centered philosophies
- Influence changes in other sectors (e.g., health insurance)

Political Action (similar to coalition advocacy, however, focuses on social change and networking, particularly to elected politicians).
- Lend support to movements that advocate for policies that are congruent with client-centered practice (e.g., the independent living movement)
- Create and broadly communicate a vision for a preferred future
- Advocate for intersectorial policy planning
- Initiate actions in a deliberate attempt to influence private and public policy choices and decisions
- Talk and write to politicians about the benefits of client-centered practice and the need for supports (e.g., time, policy changes, education) required to implement this approach

Restall, G., Stern M., & Ripat, J. *The Client-Centred Process Evaluation.* © 1997.

SECTION 5 OF 5
ACTION PLAN

Remember to detail specific objectives, actions, settings or locations, other involved individuals, and time frame when developing your action plan.

Priority	Action Plan	Time Frame

appendix d

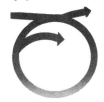

THE OCCUPATIONAL PERFORMANCE PROCESS MODEL HIGHLIGHTS

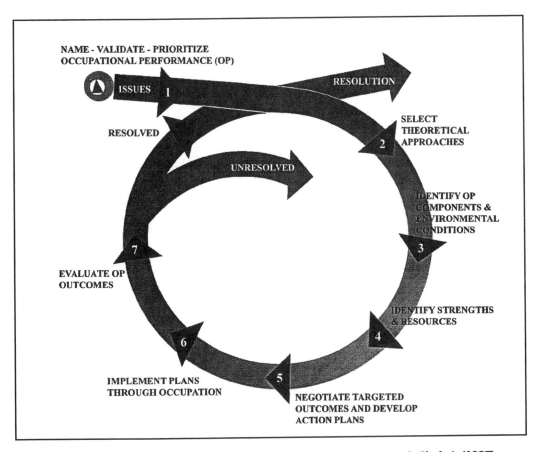

Occupational Performance Process Model. From Fearing, V.G., Law, M., & Clark, J. (1997). An occupational performance process model: Fostering client and therapist alliances. *Canadian Journal of Occupational Therapy, 64*, 11. Reprinted with permission of CAOT Publications.

STAGE 1

- Listen to client narration in context
- Focus on occupation
- Identify OPIs
- Validate and prioritize issues
- Evaluate occupational performance (OPIs) to create a baseline for use in outcome measurement

STAGE 2

- Select potential theoretical approaches related to occupation, person, and environment as fit within the context of the client's story
- Select theoretical approaches to drive subsequent assessments and interventions

STAGE 3

- Use additional assessments to investigate possible personal components or environmental conditions that may be contributing to the OPIs
- Observe relevant occupations in environments that make sense (context)
- Ensure assessments fit within the client's story
- Explain results of formal and informal assessment findings to clients through ongoing, jargon-free discussion
- Formulate and validate the problem list with the client

STAGE 4

- Use formal and informal tools to gather information regarding client strengths in person and occupation and resources in his or her environment
- Consider the strengths and resources therapists bring to the client-therapist partnership
- Consider whether the therapist has the necessary knowledge and skill to positively influence change
- Integrate this information into the intervention plan as appropriate

STAGE 5

- Determine the client's targeted outcome or vision of desired future performance related to OPIs
- Set targeted outcomes for each OPI
- Write targeted outcomes in behavioral terms and assign time frames for purposes of measurement
- Develop action plans based on all possible interventions in person, environment, and occupation that may positively influence the outcome
- Explain and negotiate interventions with clients
- Place the "what" of the action plan in order of necessary accomplishment with interventions in person generally first; then determine partnerships or the "who" of the plan and assign time frames

STAGE 6

- Confirm the "when," "where," and "how" of the plan with all parties and begin the intervention
- Monitor and document progress
- Problem-solve possible lack of progress in partnership with the client, keep in mind the balance between content and process in this intervention phase, and be flexible
- Celebrate success and support grief related to potential frustration, fear, or loss
- Facilitate seamless transition of clients and documentation to other settings for continuation of the plan as required

STAGE 7

- Measure client-specific targeted outcomes that are based in occupation
- Compare pre- and post-intervention measures
- Modify targets or identify additional goal areas as required
- Use individualized client outcomes collectively for program outcomes
- Use formal, reliable, and valid outcome measurement tools to provide the most useful information
- Use outcome measurement tools that make sense to stakeholders and are user-friendly for clients and therapists alike

GLOSSARY OF ACRONYMS

ADL: activities of daily living

AOTA: American Occupational Therapy Association

CAOT: Canadian Association of Occupational Therapists

CCPE: Client-Centred Process Evaluation
The CCPE encourages therapists to look at their values, beliefs, assumptions, behaviors, the therapeutic use of self, the "professional self," and their workplace.
The CCPE includes:
* Client questionnaire
* Clinician questionnaire
* Reflection summary form
* Compilation of client-centered strategies
* Action plan form (Restall, Stern, & Ripat, 1997) (See Chapter 13.)

CMOP: Canadian Model of Occupational Performance
"A 1997 conceptual framework that describes occupational therapy's view of the dynamic, interwoven relationship between persons, environment, and occupation that results in occupational performance over a person's lifespan" (CAOT, 1997, p. 180).

COPM: Canadian Occupational Performance Measure
"An individualized measure designed for use by occupational therapists to detect change in a client's self-perception of occupational performance over time" (Law, Baptiste, Carswell, McColl, Polatajko, & Pollock, 1994, p. 1). (See Chapter 3.)

GAS: Goal Attainment Scaling
A method of measuring change in client-specific goals. (See Chapter 9.)

GNP: gross national product

OPHI-II: Occupational Performance History Interview II
The OPHI-II is an assessment of a person's occupational life history in the areas of work, leisure, and daily life activities (Kielhofner & Henry, 1998). (See Chapter 3.)

OPPM: Occupational Performance Process Model
The OPPM is a model of practice that guides the therapist and client through a client-centered process that begins with identification of occupational performance issues important to the client and ends with resolution of those issues.

The seven stages of the OPPM are:
- Stage 1—Name, validate, and prioritize occupational performance issues
- Stage 2—Select theoretical approaches
- Stage 3—Identify occupational performance components and environmental conditions
- Stage 4—Identify strengths and resources
- Stage 5—Negotiate targeted outcomes and develop action plans
- Stage 6—Implement plans through occupation
- Stage 7—Evaluate occupational performance outcomes

OPI: occupational performance issue

An OPI is an actual or potential issue (or problem) in the person's (or organization's) "ability to choose, organize, and satisfactorily perform meaningful occupations that are culturally defined and age-appropriate for looking after oneself, enjoying life, and contributing to the social and economic fabric of a community" (CAOT, 1997, p. 181). OPIs refer to more than one occupational performance issue.

OSA: Occupational Self Assessment

The OSA is an evaluation tool that assesses personal perception of occupational competence and the environmental influences on occupational adaptation. (See Chapter 3.)

PEO: Person-Environment-Occupation model

The PEO "describes interactions beetween person, occupation, and environment" (Law, Cooper, Strong, Stewart, Rigby, & Letts, 1996, p. 9).

SAFER: Safety Assessment of Function and the Environment for Rehabilitation

The SAFER identifies environmental conditionals specific to a client's home and the interaction between the client's performance and home environment. (See Chapter 5.)

SNF: skilled nursing facility

COMPILED LIST OF REFERENCES

American Occupational Therapy Association (1999). Health coverage lost as families leave welfare. *OT Week, 31*(21), i-iii.

Arrien, A. (1993). *The four-fold way: Walking the paths of the warrior, teacher, healer and visionary.* San Francisco: Harper.

Baron, K., & Curtin, C. (1990). *Self-assessmment of occupational functioning.* Chicago: Model of Human Occupation Clearing House.

Baron, K., Kielhofner, G., Goldhammer, T., & Wolenski, J. (1999). *The Occupational Self Assessment user's manual.* Chicago: University of Chicago.

Batten, J. (1998). Servant-leadership: A passion to serve. In L.C. Spears (Ed.), *Insights on Leadership: Service, Stewardship, Spirit, and Servant-Leadership.* Toronto, Ontario, Canada: John Wiley & Sons, Inc.

Baum, C. (1980). Occupational therapists put care in the health system. *American Journal of Occupational Therapy, 34,* 505-516.

Bender, P.U. (with Hellman, E.) (1997). *Leadership from within.* Toronto, Ontario, Canada: Stoddart Publishing Co. Ltd.

Benson, H. (1997). *Timeless healing: The power and biology of belief.* New York: Fireside.

Bergmann, H., Hurson, K., & Russ-Eft, D. (1999). *Everyone a leader: A grassroots model for the new workplace.* New York: John Wiley & Sons, Inc.

Block, P. (1987). *The empowered manager* (pp. 108-116). San Francisco: Jossey-Bass Publishers.

Bosch, J. (1995). *The reliability and validity of the Canadian Occupational Performance Measure.* Unpublished master's thesis. McMaster University, Hamilton, Ontario, Canada.

Bridle, M.J., & Bell, E.B. (1975). Community placements. *Canadian Journal of Occupational Therapy, 42*(1), 13-15.

Brown, C., & Bowen, R. (1998). Including consumer and environment in occupational therapy treatment planning. *Occupational Therapy Journal of Research, 18,* 44-62.

Cadman, D., Chambers, L., Feldman, W., & Sackett, D. (1984). Assessing the effectiveness of community screening program. *Journal of the American Medical Association, 251,* 1580-1585.

Canadian Association of Occupational Therapists (CAOT) (1981). *Guidelines for the client-centred practice of occupational therapy.* Toronto, Ontario, Canada: CAOT Publications.

Canadian Association of Occupational Therapists (CAOT) (1991). *Occupational therapy guidelines for client-centred practice.* Toronto, Ontario, Canada: CAOT Publications ACE.

Canadian Association of Occupational Therapists (1994). *Occupational therapy guidelines for client-centred mental health practice.* Toronto, Ontario, Canada: CAOT Publications ACE.

Canadian Association of Occupational Therapists (1996). Profile of occupational therapy practice in Canada. *Canadian Journal of Occupational Therapy, 63,* 79-113.

Canadian Association of Occupational Therapists (CAOT) (1997). *Enabling occupation: An occupational therapy perspective.* Ottawa, Ontario, Canada: CAOT Publications ACE.

Canadian Association of Occupational Therapists (CAOT). (1999). Promotional campaign slogan. (Adapted from Wilcock, 1998.)

Carlson, J. (1996). Evaluating patient motivation in physical disabilities practice settings. *American Journal of Occupational Therapy, 51,* 347-351.

Carson, R. (1999). Client-centred practice in an American acute care rehabilitation hospital: A case study. *Occupational Therapy Now, 1*(3), 5-7.

Cassidy, D. (1999). Measuring outcomes. *Recovery, 10,* 15-17.

Cassidy, J.C., & Kolodner, E.L. (1999). Assisted living 101: Profile of a growth industry. *Gerontology Special Interest Section Quarterly, 22*(June), 1-4.

Chewning, B., & Sleath, B. (1996). Medication decision-making and management: A client-centred model. *Social Science and Medicine, 42,* 389-398.

Clark, F.A., Azen, S.P., Zemke, R., Hackson, J., Carleson, M., Mandel, D., Hay, J., Josepheson, K., Cherry, B., Hessel, C., Palmer, J., & Lipson, L. (1997). Occupational therapy for independent-living older adults: A randomized controlled trial. *Journal of the American Medical Association, 278*(6), 1321-1326.

Corring, D., & Cook, J. (1999). Client-centred care means that I am a valued human being. *Canadian Journal of Occupational Therapy, 66,* 71-82.

Covey, S.R. (1998). Foreword. In L.C. Spears (Ed.), *Insights on Leadership: Service, Stewardship, Spirit, and Servant-Leadership*. Toronto, Ontario, Canada: John Wiley & Sons, Inc.

Coyne, I. (1996). Parent participation: A concept analysis. *Journal of Advanced Nursing, 23*, 733-740.

de Clive-Lowe, S. (1996). Outcome measurement, cost-effectiveness and clinical audit: The importance of standardised assessment to occupational therapists in meeting these new demands. *British Journal of Occupational Therapy, 59*, 357-362.

Donabedian, A. (1988). The quality of care: How can it be assessed? *Journal of the American Medical Association, 260*, 1743-1748.

Dunn, W., Brown, C., & McGuigan, A. (1994). The ecology of human performance: A framework for considering the effect of context. *American Journal of Occupational Therapy, 48*, 595-607.

Egan, M., Dubouloz, C.J., von Zweck, C., & Vallerand, J. (1998). The client-centred evidence-based practice of occupational therapy. *Canadian Journal of Occupational Therapy, 65*, 136-142.

Egan, M., Warren, S.A., Hessel, P.A., & Gilewich, G. (1992). Activities of daily living following hip fracture. *Occupational Therapy Journal of Research, 12*, 342-356.

Engel, G. (1977). The need for a new medical model: A challenge for biomedicine. *Science, 196*, 129-136.

Fearing, V.G. (1993). Occupational therapists chart a course through the health record. *Canadian Journal of Occupational Therapy, 60*, 232-240.

Fearing, V.G., & Clark, J. (1998). *Reflecting on personal leadership behaviors*. Unpublished raw data.

Fearing, V.G., Clark, J., & Stanton, S. (1998). The client-centred occupational therapy process. In M. Law (Ed.), *Client-Centered Occupational Therapy*. Thorofare, NJ: SLACK Incorporated.

Fearing, V.G., Law, M., & Clark, J. (1997). An occupational performance process model: Fostering client and therapist alliances. *Canadian Journal of Occupational Therapy, 64*, 7-15.

Ferguson-Paré, M. (1998). Nursing leadership and autonomous professional practice of registered nurses. *Canadian Journal of Nursing Administration, 11*(2), 7-30.

Fleming, M. (1991). The therapist with the three-track mind. *American Journal of Occupational Therapy, 45*, 1007-1014.

Fulmer, C. (1993). Developing a reflective practice of professional development. *School Business Affairs, September*, 23-26.

Gerteis, M., Edgman-Levitan, S., Daley, J., & Delbanco, T. (Eds.). (1993). *Through the patient's eyes: Understanding and promoting patient-centred care*. San Francisco: Jossey-Bass.

Gitlin, L., Corcoran, M., & Leinmiller-Eckhardt, S. (1995). Understanding the family perspective: An ethnographic framework for providing occupational therapy in the home. *American Journal of Occupational Therapy, 49*, 802-809.

Goldstein, J. (1976). *The experience of insight*. Boston: Shambhala Publications, Inc.

Greenberger, D., & Padesky, C. (1995). *Mind over mood*. New York: Guilford Press.

Gwin, C. (1999). AOTA Southeast Regional Program Update. *OT Practice, 4*(6), 57.

Hamilton, B.B., Granger, C.V., Sherwin, F.S., Zielezny, M., & Tashman, J.S. (1987). A uniform national data system for medical rehabilitation. In M.J. Fuhrer (Ed.), *Rehabilitation Outcomes: Analysis and Measurement* (pp. 137-147). Baltimore: Paul H. Brookes.

Health Canada (1997). *National health expenditures in Canada, 1975-1996*. http://www.hc-sc.gc.ca/datapcb/datahesa/E_expend.htm

Hobson, S. (1996). Being client-centred when the client is cognitively impaired. *Canadian Journal of Occupational Therapy, 63*, 133-137.

Holden, R. (1990). Models, muddles and medicine. *International Journal of Nursing Studies, 27*, 223-234.

Hooper, B. (1997). The relationship between pretheoretical assumptions and clinical reasoning. *American Journal of Occupational Therapy, 51*, 328-338.

Iwama, M. (1999). Cross-cultural perspectives on client-centred occupational therapy practice: A view from Japan. *Occupational Therapy Now, Nov/Dec*, 4-6.

Kalmanson, B., & Seligman, S. (1992). Family-provider relationships: The basis of all interventions. *Infants and Young Children, 4*, 46-52.

Keith, R.A., Granger, C.V., Hamilton, B.B., & Sherwin, F.S. (1987). The Functional Independence Measure: A new tool for rehabilitation. In M.G. Eisenberg & R.C. Grzesiak (Eds.), *Advances in Clinical Rehabilitation* (Vol. 1, pp. 6-18). New York: Springer-Verlag.

Kielhofner, G. (1985). *A model of human occupation: Theory and applications*. Baltimore: Williams & Wilkins.

Kielhofner, G., & Henry, A. (1988). Development and investigation of the Occupational Performance History Interview. *American Journal of Occupational Therapy, 42,* 489-498.

Kielhofner, G., Mallinson, T., Crawford, D., Nowak, M., Rigby, M., Henry, A., & Walens, D. (1998). *Occupational Performance History Interview (OPHI-II).* Bethesda, MD: American Occupational Therapy Association.

King, S., Rosenbaum, P., & King, G. (1996). Parent's perceptions of caregiving: Development and validation of a measure of processes. *Developmental Medicine and Child Neurology, 38,* 757-772.

Kiresuck, T.J., & Sherman, R.E. (1968). Goal attainment scaling: A general method for evaluating comprehensive community mental health programs. *Community Mental Health Journal, 4,* 443-453.

Klein, E., & Izzo, J.B. (1999). *Awakening corporate soul: Four paths to unleashing the power of people at work.* Lions Bay, British Columbia, Canada: Fairwinds Press.

Kouzes, J.M. (1998). Finding your voice. In L.C. Spears (Ed.), *Insights on Leadership: Service, Stewardship, Spirit, and Servant-Leadership.* Toronto, Ontario, Canada: John Wiley & Sons, Inc.

Law, M. (1991). The environment: A focus for occupational therapy. *Canadian Journal of Occupational Therapy, 58*(4), 171-179.

Law, M. (Ed.). (1998). *Client-centered occupational therapy.* Thorofare, NJ: SLACK Incorporated.

Law, M., Baptiste, S., Carswell, A., McColl, M.A., Polatajko, H., & Pollock, N. (1994). *Canadian Occupational Performance Measure manual (COPM)* (2nd ed.). Toronto, Ontario, Canada: CAOT Publications ACE.

Law, M., Baptiste, S., Carswell, A., McColl, M.A., Polatajko, H., & Pollock, N. (1998). *The Canadian Occupational Performance Measure (COPM)* (3rd ed.). Ottawa, Ontario, Canada: CAOT Publications.

Law, M., Baptiste, S., & Mills, J. (1995). Client-centred practice: What does it mean and does it make a difference? *Canadian Journal of Occupational Therapy, 62,* 250-257.

Law, M.C., Baum, C.M., & Dunn, W. (2000). *Measuring occupational performance: A guide to best practice.* Thorofare, NJ: SLACK Incorporated.

Law, M., Brown, S., Barnes, S., King, G., Rosenbaum, P., & King, S. (1997). *Implementing family-centred services in Ontario children's rehabilitation services.* Hamilton, Ontario, Canada: Neurodevelopmental Clinical Research Unit.

Law, M., Cooper, B., Strong, S., Stewart, D., Rigby, P., & Letts, L. (1996). The Person-Environment-Occupation model: A transactive approach to occupational performance. *Canadian Journal of Occupational Therapy, 63,* 9-23.

Law, M., & Mills, J. (1998). Client-centred occupational therapy. In M. Law (Ed.), *Client-Centered Occupational Therapy* (pp. 2-18). Thorofare, NJ: SLACK Incorporated.

Law, M., Polatajko, H., Pollock, N., McColl, M.A., Carswell, A., & Baptiste, S. (1994). The Canadian Occupational Performance Measure: Results of pilot testing. *Canadian Journal of Occupational Therapy, 61,* 191-197.

Law, M., & Stewart, D. (1996). *Test retest reliability of the COPM with children.* Unpublished manuscript. McMaster University School of Rehabilitation Science, Hamilton, Ontario, Canada.

Letts, L., Scott, S., Burtney, J., Marshall, L., & McKean, M. (1998). The reliability and validity of the Safety Assessment of Function and the Environment for Rehabilitation (SAFER) tool. *British Journal of Occupational Therapy, 61,* 127-132.

MacKenzie, G. (1996). *Orbiting the giant hairball: A corporate fool's guide to surviving with grace.* Toronto, Ontario, Canada: Penguin Books, Ltd.

Matheson, L. (1998). Engaging the person in the process: Planning together for occupational therapy intervention. In M. Law (Ed.), *Client-Centered Occupational Therapy* (pp. 108-119). Thorofare, NJ: SLACK Incorporated.

Mattingly, C. (1991). The narrative nature of clinical reasoning. *American Journal of Occupational Therapy, 45,* 998-1005.

McColl, M.A. (1998). What do we need to know to practice occupational therapy in the community? *American Journal of Occupational Therapy, 52*(1), 11-18.

McColl, M.A., Law, M., & Stewart, D. (1992). *Theoretical basis of occupational therapy.* Thorofare, NJ: SLACK Incorporated.

McColl, M.A., Patterson, M., Doubt, L., & Law, M. (In press). Validation of the COPM for community practice. *Canadian Journal of Occupational Therapy.*

Mew, M., & Fossey, E. (1996). Client-centred aspects of clinical reasoning during an initial assessment using the Canadian Occupational Performance Measure. *Australian Occupational Therapy Journal, 43,* 155-166.

Mirkopoulos, C., & Butler, K. (1994). *Quality assurance: Clients' perceptions of goal performance and satisfaction.* Proceedings of the 11th World Congress of Occupational Therapy. London, England.

Neistadt, M.E. (1987). An occupational therapy program for adults with developmental disabilities. *American Journal of Occupational Therapy, 41,* 433-438.

Neistadt, M.E. (1995). Methods of assessing clients' priorities: A survey of adult physical dysfunction settings. *American Journal of Occupational Therapy, 49,* 428-436.

Neistadt, M.E., & Marques, K. (1984). An independent living skills training program. *American Journal of Occupational Therapy, 38,* 671-676.

Novartis Foundation for Gerontological Research (1999). *Putting age on hold: Delaying the diseases of old age.* http://www.healthandage.com/publi/0108020023/page2.htm.

Oliver, R., Blathwayt, J., Brackley, C., & Tamaki, T. (1993). Development of the Safety Assessment of Function and the Environment for Rehabilitation (SAFER) tool. *Canadian Journal of Occupational Therapy, 60,* 78-82.

O'Neil, J. (1997). *Leadership Aikido: 6 business practices to turn around your life.* New York: Harmony Books.

Pollock, N., & McColl, M.A. (1998). Assessment in client-centred occupational therapy. In M. Law (Ed.), *Client-Centered Occupational Therapy.* Thorofare, NJ: SLACK Incorporated.

Polya, G. (1957). *How to solve it* (2nd ed.). Garden City, NY: Doubleday Anchor Books.

Price-Lackey, P., & Cashman, J. (1996). Jenny's story: Reinventing oneself through occupation and narrative configuration. *American Journal of Occupational Therapy, 50,* 306-314.

Rackow, B. (1996). *Priority Intervention Criteria.* Unpublished raw data.

Rebeiro, K., & Miller Polgar, J. (1999). Enabling occupational performance: Optimal experiences in therapy. *Canadian Journal of Occupational Therapy, 66,* 14-22.

Reed, K.L. (1984). *Models of practice in occupational therapy.* Baltimore: Williams & Wilkins.

Registered Nurses Association of British Columbia (1992). *Determinants of health: Empowering strategies for nursing practice.* Vancouver, British Columbia, Canada: Author.

Restall, G., & Stern, M. (1996, April). *Being client-centred in a medical model environment.* Short course presented at the annual meeting of the American Occupational Therapy Association, Chicago.

Restall, G., Stern, M., & Ripat, J. (1997). *The client-centred process evaluation.* Unpublished document.

Rizzo, J. (1993). Physician uncertainty and the art of persuasion. *Social Science and Medicine, 37,* 1451-1459.

Robinson, V.M. (1991). *Humor and the health professions: The therapeutic use of humor in health care* (2nd ed.). Thorofare, NJ: SLACK Incorporated.

Rockwood, K., Joyce, B., & Stolee, P. (1997). Use of Goal Attainment Scaling in measuring clinically important change in cognitive rehabilitation patients. *Journal of Clinical Epidemiology, 50,* 581-588.

Rockwood, K., Stolee, P., & Fox, R.A. (1993). Use of Goal Attainment Scaling in measuring clinically important change in the frail elderly. *Journal of Clinical Epidemiology, 46,* 1113-1118.

Rogers, C. (1957). The necessary and sufficient conditions of therapeutic personality change. *Journal of Consulting Psychology, 21*(2), 95-103.

Ross, R.B. (1994). The ladder of inference. In P.M. Senge, A. Kleiner, C Roberts, R.B. Ross, & B.J. Smith. *The Fifth Discipline Fieldbook: Strategies and Tools for Building a Learning Organization* (pp. 242-246). New York: Doubleday.

Ryden, M., & Rustad, R. (1985). Wellness model replaces medical model. *Journal of Long-Term Care Administration, 13,* 115-119.

Sackett, D., Haynes, B., Tugwell, P., & Guyatt, G. (1996). *Clinical epidemiology.* Oxford, England: Oxford Press.

Sanford, J., Law, M., Swanson, L., & Guyatt, G. (1994). *Assessing clinically important change as an outcome of rehabilitation in older adults.* Paper presented at the Conference of the American Society of Aging, San Francisco.

Schaef, A.W. (1996). *Meditations for women who do too much.* New York: HarperCollins.

Schaef, A.W. (1998). *Living in process: Basic truths for living the path of the soul.* Toronto, Ontario, Canada: Random House.

Schell, B., & Cervero, R. (1993). Clinical reasoning in occupational therapy: An integrative review. *American Journal of Occupational Therapy, 47,* 605-610.

Schön, D. (1983). *The reflective practitioner: How professionals think in action.* New York: Basic Books.

Schön, D. (1987). *Educating the reflective practitioner.* San Francisco: Jossey-Bass.

Scott Lee, S.J. (1999). Lobbying for occupational therapy. *OT Practice, 4*(8), 5-12.

Senge, P.M. (1990a). *The fifth discipline: The art and practice of the learning organization* (pp. 64-65). New York: Doubleday.

Senge, P.M. (1990b). The leader's new work: Building learning organizations. *Sloane Management Review, 32*(1), 9.

Senge, P., Roberts, C., Rosser, B., Smith, B.J., & Kleiner, A. (1994). *The fifth discipline fieldbook*. New York: Doubleday.

Shaeffer, J. (1996). *The stone people: Living together in a different world*. Waterloo, Ontario, Canada: Forsyth Publications.

Sherr-Klein, B. (1997). *Slow dance A story of stroke, love and disability*. Toronto, Ontario, Canada: Random House.

Siebert, C. (1999). Meeting the challenge of new home health care mandates. *OT Practice, 4*(2), 25-29.

Smith, J.S. (1990). *Patenting the sun: Polio and the Salk vaccine*. New York: William Morrow and Co., Inc.

Smyth, C.J., Freyberg, R.H., & McEwen, C. (1985). *History of rheumatology*. Atlanta: Arthritis Foundation.

Spencer, J., & Davidson, H. (1998). The Community Adaptive Planning Assessment: A clinical tool for documenting future planning with clients. *American Journal of Occupational Therapy, 52*, 19-30.

Spencer, J., Davidson, H., & White, V. (1997). Helping clients develop hopes for the future. *American Journal of Occupational Therapy, 51*, 191-198.

Spencer, J., Krefting, L., & Mattingly, C. (1993). Incorporation of ethnographic methods in occupational therapy assessment. *American Journal of Occupational Therapy, 47*, 303-309.

Stanton, S., Kramer, C., & Thompson-Franson, T. (1997). Linking concepts to a process for organizing occupational therapy services. In Canadian Association of Occupational Therapists, *Enabling Occupation: An Occupational Therapy Perspective*. Ottawa, Ontario, Canada: CAOT Publications.

Statistics Canada. (1997, June). CANSIM database: Canadian socio-economic information management system http://www/datalib./finance/cansim/cansite.htm.

Statistics Canada, Health Canada, Division for Aging and Seniors. (1999). *Canada's Seniors-No. 37: Life expectancy rising and No. 12: Living in Institutions*.

Steinem, G. (1992). *Revolution from within: A book of self-esteem*. Toronto, Ontario, Canada: Little, Brown & Co.

Stern, M., & Restall, G. (1993, June). *Client-centred practice and the medical model*. Paper presented at the annual meeting of the Canadian Association of Occupational Therapists, Regina, Saskatchewan, Canada.

Stoch, D. (1999). Identifying the client: The challenge of client-centred practice in a fee-for-service system. *Occupational Therapy Now, March/April*, 8-9.

Stolee, P., Rockwood, K., Fox, R.A., & Streiner, D.L. (1992). The use of Goal Attainment Scaling in a geriatric care setting. *Journal of the American Geriatrics Society, 40*, 574-578.

Stricoff, R. (1999). The evolution of a solo practitioner's role as a rehabilitation ergonomist within a large corporation. *Work Programs Special Interest Section Quarterly, 13*, 2.

Strong, S., Rigby, P., Stewart, D., Law, M., Letts, L., & Cooper, B. (1999). Application of the Person-Environment-Occupation model: A practical tool. *Canadian Journal of Occupational Therapy, 66*, 122-133.

Sumsion, T. (1993). Client-centred practice: The true impact. *Canadian Journal of Occupational Therapy, 60*, 6-8.

Townsend, E., Stanton, S., Law, M., Polatajko, H., Baptiste, S., Thompson-Franson, T., Kramer, C., Swedlove, F., Brintnell, S., & Campanile, L. (1997). *Enabling occupation: An occupational therapy perspective*. Ottawa, Ontario, Canada: CAOT Publications.

Turner, A. (1996). The philosophy and history of occupational therapy. In A. Turner, M. Foster, & S.E. Johnson (Eds.), *Occupational Therapy and Physical Dysfunction* (4th ed., pp. 3-25). London: Churchill Livingstone.

Ware, J.E., Phillips, J., Yody, B.B., & Adamczyk, J. (1996). Assessment tools: Functional health status and patient satisfaction. *American Journal of Medical Quality, 11*, S50-S53.

Webster's Third New International Dictionary of the English Language Unabridged. (1981). Springfield, MA: Merriam-Webster.

Whyte, D. (1994). *The heart aroused*. New York: Doubleday.

Wilcock, A.A. (1998). Reflections on doing, being and becoming. *Canadian Journal of Occupational Therapy, 65*, 248-256.

Wilcox, A. (1994). *A study of verbal guidance for children with developmental coordination disorder*. Unpublished master's thesis. University of Western Ontario, London, Ontario.

Wilson, M. (1999). Client self-referral: Starting the process right. *Occupational Therapy Now, January/February*, 22-24.

Wood-Dauphinee, S., Arsenault, A.B., & Richards, C.L. (1994). Outcome assessment in rehabilitation. Overview of the 2nd National Rehabilitation Conference. *Canadian Journal of Rehabilitation, 7*, 171-184.

Wythenshawe Hospital Manchester (1999). *Interesting facts about transplantation*. http://www.nh-ns.man.ac.uk/NHNSpics.htm.

Yerxa, E. (1980). Occupational therapy's role in creating a future climate of caring. *American Journal of Occupational Therapy, 34*, 529-534.

INDEX